'When diet is wrong, medicine is of no use. When diet is correct, medicine is of no need.'

Ayurvedic Wisdom

There are numerous disorders that can be prevented and treated by eating natural foods rich in minerals, vitamins, trace elements, vital nutrients and other substances which have positive medicinal properties.

Examples abound: The ancients knew that apple cleansed the blood, controlled high blood pressure and stimulated the flow of urine. Now, science has validated this. Apples lower sodium chloride, increase potassium and body's alkaline reserves.

Medical research has established onion as an effective preventive against heart disease; they correct thrombosis and reduce blood cholesterol. Garlic juice dissolves accumulated mucus in the sinus cavities, bronchial tubes, lungs and reduces the severity of asthmatic attacks. Blood sugar is controlled by *amla*; it stimulates production of insulin.

Scurvy resists treatment with synthetic vitamin C, yet responds quickly to certain vegetables and fruit like cabbage, lemon and limes. The list is endless...

Lucid, easy-to-follow and devoid of medical jargon, the book is an invaluable guide for a better understanding of health, food and natural remedies.

Eat healthy. Live healthier.

The Author

H.K. Bakhru enjoys countrywide reputation as an expert naturopath and a writer on the subject. His well researched articles on nature cure, health and nutrition appear regularly in the media.

A diploma holder in naturopathy, he is a member of the Nature Cure Practitioners' Guild in Mumbai. He has made extensive study on naturopathy and herbalism. He spends his retired life propagating and practising nature cure and is always willing to offer advice to those who seek his help.

His other books, all bestsellers, are *Herbs That Heal, Vitamins That Heal, Natural Home Remedies for Common Ailments,* and *Conquering Diabetes Naturally.*

'His books are read all world over; his forte is nature cure, a much sought after alternative to allopathic medicine. He is acknowledged as an expert on the topic.'

Times of India

FOODS THAT HEAL

The Natural Way to Good Health

H.K. Bakhru

Orient Paperbacks
DELHI | MUMBAI

Acknowledgments

I am grateful to Dr. J.M. Jussawalla, an eminent naturopath and a member of the Governing Body of the Central Council of Research in Yoga and Naturopathy for this foreword.

Disclaimer

The information in this book is general in nature and for reference and guidance only. It is not a substitute for medical advice and the readers are urged to consult their doctor before taking decisions which are medical in nature.

Editors: Ananda Iyer/S Malhotra

www.orientpaperbacks.in

ISBN : 978-81-222-0720-0

Foods That Heal: The Natural Way to Good Health

Subject: Health & Fitness / Herbal / Natural Medicine

1st Published 1990
2nd Rev & Enlarged Edition 2022
This Printing 2025

Published by
Orient Paperbacks
(A division of Vision Books Pvt. Ltd.)
5A/8 Ansari Road, New Delhi-110 002

Cover design by Vision Studio

Printed and bound at Saurabh Printers, Noida

FOREWORD

Never before has an average person been better fed yet so poorly nourished. There is an increasing concentration of population in cities, metropolis, and megapolis. As a consequence we have become divorced from nature and its beautiful bounty. Innumerable preserved, refrigerated, treated, processed, chemicalized and pasteurized food items are promoted twenty four-seven for making them a commercial success. Such foods can never substitute wholesome, natural food.

Undoubtedly, this advertisement driven culture has denied the present generation of farm-fresh, nutritious natural foods. Most food, specially the increasingly popular 'convenience foods' are largely denatured, artificially flavoured, turgid, semi-synthetic and devoid of their vital food values. Whatever nutrients are left in them after processing, storage and transportation are poor substitutes for natural "wholesomeness". Such packaged and preserved foods are nothing but junk food.

Foods That Heal is a valuable reference book for one and all seeking good health and prevention of ailments. This practical guide on natural foods is exhaustive study of food values, curative and natural benefits of all food items used in our every day life.

Dr. J.M. Jussawalla
Director and President,
International Federation of the
Scientific Research Society, India.
Director, Natural Therapy Clinic, Bombay.

PREFACE

'Let food be thy medicine and medicine be thy food', said Hippocrates, father of modern medicine. This maxim is more relevant today than at any time in human history. I write this from personal experience; words of Hippocrates have been prophetic in my case. I was afflicted with serious ailments at an early age. At the age of 16 years, I contracted pleurisy and typhoid fever of long duration. With age, I became afflicted with numerous ailments, including hyperacidity with severe heartburn, breathing trouble, stroke, suspected brain tumour, chronic duodenal ulcer, spondylosis, myalgia, hiatus hernia with peptic oesophageal ulcers, suspected heart disease, backache and prostate enlargement.

The medical science failed to provide any relief and I underwent both physical suffering and mental anguish for over 40 years. Eventually, I gave up all drugs and resorted to the natural healing.

Diet played a decisive role in the success of this therapy. It was primarily through a selective diet of natural foods such as fresh and dried fruits, vegetables, grains, nuts, seeds and special protective foods like milk, curd and honey that I succeeded in controlling several dreaded disabilities. The experience prompted me to explore the medicinal virtues of foods in their natural form. I popularised by findings through a series of articles in *The Times of India, The Economic Times* and other publications. The response was overwhelming. I was encouraged to study the subject in greater depth and and the result is this book about the use of natural foods in healing of specific diseases and living a healthier life.

H.K. Bakhru

Contents

> Fruits and vegetables are pure gifts from Mother Nature and the most natural way to heal your body and make yourself whole again.
>
> — Farnoosh Brock
> Int'l Speaker & Trainer

trans fat that is bad for your heart health. Olive Oil, does not offer extra benefits compared to our *sarson ka tel.*

Cabbage

Kale, a super healthy green, became an international favourite because it is loaded with vitamins and minerals. But cabbage is an equally good substitute, nutritionally at par with Kale.

Cabbage is a nutritiously rich vegetable and one which is abundant in Vitamin C. It has similar nutrition value as Kale. And we all know cabbage and love its taste.

> A healthy diet is not only a
> solution to many of our
> health problems.
> It's the most important solution.

Kuttu or Buckwheat

Buckwheat or Kuttu is a staple fasting food widely used in many parts of India, especially during *Navratri* and *Janamashtmi.* It is packed with nutrients like protein, magnesium, Vitamin E, fibre and good amounts of energy. It is rich in anti-oxidants and helps reduce bad cholesterol. It supports weight loss, lowers cholesterol and can help prevent diabetes and digestive disorders.

Buckwheat is an excellent substitute to oats, the popular breakfast cereal among those trying to lose weight.

Tea

A cup or two of tea a day can be good for your health. Tea contains few calories, helps with hydration, and is a good source of antioxidants.

A recent study, published in *European Journal of Preventive Cardiology* reported that those who drink tea regularly are less likely to develop atherosclerotic cardiovascular disease.

Tea, especially green teas, contain potent anti-oxidants, are a rich source of flavonoids, bioactive compounds that can lessen oxidative stress, relieve inflammation, and provide other health benefits.

Kala Jamun or Indian Blackberry

As Dr. Sagandh Goel says, 'Chinese Goji berries (small red berries) gained popularity for they may help stabilize blood sugar. But the *desi* alternative, *Kala Jamun* can also control blood sugar and improve immunity. It is rich in calcium potassium, iron, and vitamin C.'

Compared to Goji berry with 48 mg of vitamin C per 100 gm amla has 252 mg of vitamin C — almost 5 times! Match that!!

Ghia or Bottle Gourd

Ghia is a common, inexpensive vegetable available with your local *sabzi-wala* throughout the year. It can help you lose weight the same way as more internationally famous and popular Zucchini. Like Zucchini, it is low in calories, reduces hunger, keep your appetite at bay and help you lose weight.

So next time, be wise and buy Ghia, not Zucchini.

Sabja or Basil seeds

Sabja seeds or basil seeds, are black seeds that look a lot like chia seeds and offer immense health benefits. They are different from the holy basil, called *Tulsi.* Sabja seeds typically come from sweet basil i.e. *Qcimum basilicum,* and commonly known as sweet basil seeds. They are rich in alpha-linolenic acid and full of fibre, protein, prevent unwanted cravings, keep you full for a long time, and aid in weight loss. Surprisingly these seeds contain no calories.

The international equivalent to sabja seeds are the thrice as expensive Chia seeds with similar nutritional composition.

Mustard Oil

Mustard oil reduces inflamation, has antimicrobial properties, is abundant in Vitamin E, and is free from unhealthy cholesterol and

> 'Possibly, not all internationally available superfoods like Quinoa, Avocado, Chia Seeds, Kale are nutritionally viable for Indian bodies. That is why eating more local produce is better suited for our body type.'
>
> — *Dr. Saugandh Goel*

DESI SUPERFOODS

Foods with maximum nutritional benefits for minimal calories are referred to as "superfoods". They are packed with high amounts of micro and macro-nutrients such as vitamins, minerals, protein, fibre, Omega 3 acids, and other antioxidants.

Superfoods are not cure-all foods. A lot of people have unrealistic expectations thinking they'll be protected from chronic diseases and health problems. That is *not* correct. Superfoods have little or no value in a regimen based on unhealthy diet.

Eat a "super diet", not merely superfoods

Including superfoods is great, but only when eating a daily overall healthy and balanced diet.

Let us value the wisdom and lifestyle of our elders, and eat what our parents and grandparents recognized as healthy food.

- At only half the price
- For twice the taste
- And have similar (or even higher) nutrition value.

***Amla* or Indian gooseberries**

The humble amla is a superfood! It has twenty times more vitamin C than the internationally famous equivalent Acai or Blueberries.

It not only boosts immunity but is also known for its anti-aging and weight loss properties. Additionally, it improves brain and eye health. Although a seasonal food, it can be preserved for year round use by traditional techniques like drying, pickling, etc.

You are what you eat.
Ancient Indian proverb

FOODS THAT HEAL

Don't eat anything your grandmother wouldn't recognize as food. There are a great many food items today she wouldn't call food... stay away from these

Prof. Michael Pollan
Knight Prof. of Science & Environmental Journalism,
Univ. of California, Berkley

Index of Diseases/Ailments & Foods That Benefit

An alphabetical index of diseases, common ailments which can be prevented and healed by healthier food choices.

RED, YELLOW, GREEN, ORANGE OR... ?

That every meal should have several different colours is a good example of grandma's cookery being good science.

By picking colourful fruits and vegetables in your meal, you increase intake of important nutrients.

'Fruits and vegetables contain phytonutrients, which give them their colour, taste and aroma. These phytonutrients protect us from chronic diseases such as cancer, heart diseases, vision loss and so on' says Radhika Iyer an Ayurvedic science expert.

Dr. N. Kumar of Cancer Centre & Research Institute, University of S Florida confirms. 'Colourful food not only lowers cancer risk but also prevents the ageing process. Specific nutrients have specific colours. The deeper the colour of a food, the more of that kind of nutrients it has.'

Red is rich in lycopene which reduces cancer risks — tomatoes, watermelons, grapes, strawberries, red apples.

Orange/Yellow have amazing anti-inflammation properties e.g. turmeric. They are also rich in Vitamin C — oranges, papayas.

Yellow/Green are rich sources of carotenoids lutein and zeaxanthin which contribute to eye health — spinach, corn, amla, green peas.

Green contain sulforaphane which stimulates liver to make compounds that breakdown cancer-causing chemicals. Green plants are also full of iron and vitamins — broccoli, spinach, cabbage.

White/Brown contain allicin which has anti-tumour properties, lowers cholesterol and high blood pressure — onions, garlic, pears.

If you want to live well, you have to eat colour!

IMPORTANCE OF FRUITS IN DIET

There are numerous references to fruits in ancient literature. The *Vedas* state that fruits are the 'Food of Gods'. According to the *Quran*, fruits like grapes, dates, figs, olives and pomegranates are heavenly gifts.

In the ancient times fruits were believed to be endowed with divine properties. Fruits were revered and dedicated to gods and goddesses. Designs and shapes of various fruit were used in decorating temples, ceremonial garments and sacred vessels.

Fruits, fresh and dry, have been the a part of our staple diet. They contain substantial quantities of essential nutrients and are excellent sources of minerals, vitamins and enzymes; easily digested they also have a cleansing effect on the blood and the digestive tract. Persons subsisting on fruit diet tend to enjoy better health. Finally, fruits are not only good food but also a good medicine.

Natural Benefits of Fruits

Hydrating Effect: Fruits and fruit juices are the most pleasant way of hydrating the body. The water absorbed in this manner has an added advantage of supplying both sugar and minerals together.

Diuretic Effect: Clinical observations show that potassium, magnesium and sodium content of fruit acts as a diuretic and a diuresis — not only does the frequency of urination increase, but the urine density gets lowered and the elimination of nitrogenous waste and chlorides is accelerated. With their low level of sodium, fruit make a valuable contribution to any salt-free diet.

Alkalinising Effect: Fruit are highly beneficial in maintaining acid-alkaline balance. They neutralise the increased toxicity resulting from excessive intake of acid-forming foods and restore alkalinity. They help clear the system of morbid waste and cater to the body's requirement of natural sugar, vitamins and minerals.

The organic acids of the salts in fruit produce alkaline carbonates which alkalise the fluids. The carbohydrates of fruits are chiefly in the form of sugar, dextrin and acids which are easily digested and completely absorbed. Hence, fruit are very useful for quick energy and warmth in sickness.

Mineralising Effect: Fruit are a source of minerals. Dried fruit such as apricots, raisins and dates are rich in calcium, iron, minerals, essential for strong bones and good blood. Some fruit, like custard apple, furnish calcium to the extent of 800 mg per fruit, which is sufficient for our daily requirement.

Laxative Effect: The fibrous matter or cellulose in fruit aid in smooth passage of food through the digestive tract and promote easy bowel action. Regular use of fruits prevents constipation.

Tonic Action: Fruits exert a tonic effect in the body. Guavas, custard apples, papaya and citrus fruits, like lemons and oranges, are valuable sources of vitamin C. Several fruit contain good amounts of carotene which gets converted to vitamin A in the body. A medium-sized mango can provide as much as 15,000 international units of vitamin A which is sufficient for one week.

Fruits are at their best when eaten in their natural state, whether raw or ripe. In cooking, they lose a part of the nutrient salts and carbohydrates. They are most beneficial when taken as a separate meal or for breakfast. A combination of fruits with vegetables is not considered good. If it becomes necessary to take fruit as part of a regular meal, they should form a major portion. It is also desirable to take one kind of a fruit at a time.

In case of sickness, fruit juice should be the preferred option. However, juice should be taken immediately after extraction as it begins to decompose and loses its properties.

Vitamins, minerals, enzymes and trace elements in fresh juice are extremely beneficial in normalising body processes. They stimulate and promote body's internal healing activity and regeneration.

Curative Properties: Some fruits can combat specific ailments. It should, however, be remembered that in fruit treatment nothing except that particular fruit or its juice should be taken. Thus, when utilising lemon juice as a food remedy, the juice should be taken at least half an hour before consuming any other food.

Fruits like apple, dates and mango have a direct action on the central nervous system. Phosphorus, glutamic acid and vitamins A and B-complex of these fruit exert a protective tonic effect on the nerves. Their regular consumption sharpens memory and prevents nervous exhaustion, mental tension, hysteria and insomnia.

All berries, being extremely rich in iron, phosphorus and sodium, are highly beneficial for blood and the nerves. Lemon is a good food remedy for liver ailments, indigestion and rheumatism. Watermelons make the best kidney cleansers. The water flushes through the kidneys and the traces of various minerals contained in the water act as healing agents.

Pineapple and pomegranates are helpful in catarrh, hay fever and other chronic nasal and bronchial problems. The common cold may be treated with grapefruit juice. It helps to get rid of any infection by activating the organs of elimination.

Fresh, fully ripe fruits like grapes, apples, bananas and figs are best suited for brain deficiencies. They contain a superior quality of easily assimilable sugar which is transformed into physical energy that refreshes the brain. The kernel of walnut is a positive remedy for weakness of the brain.

A generous intake of fruit prevents disease and keep a person energetic and active even in old age.

APPLE

Botanical Name: *Malus sylvestris*
Indian Name: *Seb or Sev*

Apple is one of the most valuable of all fruit. Scandinavians called it the "Food of Gods" and believed that it had medicinal properties to regenerate mind and body.

Apple is a sub-acid, fleshy fruit with tough skin, ranging in colour from greenish yellow to red. It is usually five to seven cms in diameter with a pinkish or yellowish white flesh.

It is considered a "protective" and a wholesome food. Apart from its energy value, it plays an important role in normal development of metabolic functions i.e. the chemical and physical changes that take place within the body and enable its continued growth and functioning.

Origin and Distribution: Apple is a native of Eastern Europe and Western Asia. It is mentioned in the annals of old China, Babylon and Egypt; the Bible also contains several references to this fruit. In India, apples are grown in Kashmir, Kulu, Kumaon and Himachal. Nearly 7,500 varieties of the fruit are grown the world over.

Food Value: Apple is a highly nutritive food, rich in minerals and vitamins. Its food value is chiefly because of its sugar content which ranges from 9 to 51 per cent. Of this, fruit sugar constitutes 60 per cent, glucose 25 per cent and cane sugar only 15 per cent.

Raw apples generally contain a small quantity of starch which gets wholly converted into sugar during the process of ripening. The acid content of apple also increases with sugar. The acid constituent, mostly malic acid, is fully utilised by the body.

Natural Benefits and Curative Properties

There is an old proverb which says 'to eat an apple before going to bed will make the doctor beg his bread'. The modern version of this saying, 'an apple a day keeps the doctor away', sums up the nourishing qualities of the fruit.

Apple *

Food Value		Minerals and Vitamins	
Moisture	84.6%	Calcium	10 mg
Protein	0.2%	Phosphorus	14 mg
Fat	0.5%	Iron	1 mg
Minerals	0.3%	Vitamin A	40 IU**
Fibre	1.0%	Small amounts of	
Carbohydrates	13.4%	Vitamin E, H & B Complex	
	100%		

**Values per 100 gms edible portion | Calorific Value - 59 | **Int'l Unit*

The active medicinal principle of apple is pectin, a natural therapeutic ingredient in the inner portion of the rind and the pulp. Pectin aids in detoxification by supplying 'galacturonic acid' needed for elimination of certain harmful substances. The malic acid in the apple is beneficial for bowels, liver and brain.

Anaemia

Apples, being rich in iron, arsenic and phosphorus, are highly beneficial in treating anaemia. Fresh apple juice is particularly recommended. Juice of upto 1 kg of apples can be taken daily with beneficial results. The best time to take juice is half an hour before meals and just before retiring to bed. The cider should be drawn from thoroughly washed apples.

Constipation and Diarrhoea

Apples are beneficial in treating both constipation and diarrhoea. Raw apples are good for constipation. At least two apples should be taken daily for proper bowel evacuation. Cooked or baked apples are good for diarrhoea. Cooking softens the cellulose and provides bulk to faeces.

Dysentery

The American Medical Association advocates the use of apples as a therapeutic agent in dysentery amongst children. Pulp of ripe and sweet apples maybe given several times a day, in quantities from one to four tablespoonfuls, according to age.

Stomach Disorders

A natural 'apple medicine' for upset stomach is prepared by slicing a whole apple and pounding it gently until it becomes slightly mashed. The mashed apple, except for the stem and seeds, may be sprinkled with cinnamon or honey and chewed thoroughly. This 'natural medicine' should be taken several times between meals. Pectin in mashed apple works to create a protective coating by virtue of its absorbent and a demulcent qualities.

Taken before meals, shredded apple mixed with a tablespoonful of honey and sprinkled with sesame seeds, constitutes an excellent stomach tonic and an appetiser. It stimulates the digestive juices and facilitates assimilation of food for healthful results.[1]

Headache

A ripe apple, after removing the upper rind and the inner hard portion, with a little salt is recommended every morning on empty stomach. This should be for a week even in chronic headache.

Heart Disease

Apples are rich in potassium and phosphorus but low in sodium. From the ancient times, apple with honey has been considered an effective remedy for functional disorders of the heart. Research by Dr. Elizabeth Barret-Cannor of California University revealed that people who consume plenty of potassium through food are likely to escape heart attacks. As a good source of potassium apples help in alleviating heart disease.

High Blood Pressure/Hypertension

Apple diet has a rapid and considerable diuretic effect causing increased secretion of urine and thus bringing down blood pressure. It also relieves the kidneys by reducing the supply of sodium chloride to a minimum. In addition, the high level of potassium in apples lowers the sodium level in the tissues.

Rheumatic Afflictions

Apples make an excellent food medicine for gout, arthritis and rheumatism especially when these diseases are caused by uric acid poisoning. The malic acid neutralises the uric acid thus affording relief. Apples, boiled to a jelly, make a very good liniment for

1. Carlson Wade, *Health Secrets from the Orient*, pp. 62-63, Allied Publishers Pvt. Ltd., Bombay.

rheumatic pains. This jelly can be rubbed freely on the affected areas.

Dry Cough

Sweet apples are valuable in dry hacking cough. Nearly 250 gms of sweet apples should be taken daily for about a week.

Kidney Stones

In countries where natural unsweetened cider is a common beverage, cases of stone or calculus are practically absent.

Eye Disorders

Apple peel water is an excellent medicine for the inflamed eyes — both as a beverage and as an eye wash. The beverage is prepared by putting the peelings in a pan with water, brought to a boiling point and allowed to simmer for a few minutes. The water is then strained and some honey be added to it.[1]

Over-ripe apples are useful as a poultice for sore eyes The pulp is applied over the closed eyes and held in position with a bandage for one to two hours.

Dental Disorders

In his book *Dental Survey,* Dr. T.T. Hanks says, 'Apples have a mouth cleansing property that no other fruit possesses, and taken after meals, they have the same effect as brushing your teeth with the added advantage that the acid content promotes the flow of saliva which is also beneficial to the teeth'[2]. The acid of the apple also exerts an antiseptic influence on the germs present in the mouth and on the teeth when thoroughly chewed. Apples are thus a natural preserver of teeth and advised in all tooth troubles.

Promotes Vigour and Vitality

Apples contain more phosphorus and iron than any other fruit or vegetable. This makes them almost an ideal fruit to tone up a weak and run-down condition. Regular consumption of apples with milk

---

1. Eric F.W. Powell, *Health from the Kitchen*, p. 22, Health Science Press, England.
2. Dr. S.J. Singh, *Food Remedies*, p. 21, Nature Cure Council of Medical Research, Lucknow, 1982.

promotes health and youthfulness and acts as an aid for a healthy and bright skin. It also has a calming, relaxing effect and is good especially for sedentary workers.

Uses

Apple is generally taken raw and is often used as a dessert or in fruit salad. It can also be cooked or baked. Apples can be used as dried apple, apple jelly, apple juice or cider and vinegar. Fresh apple juice is one of the best fruit juices.

Precautions: Apples are often sprayed with poisonous chemicals to prevent decay and should be thoroughly washed before consumption.

Don't Peel the Skin Off !

Peeling the skin off an apple means throwing away the fibre. Almost half the vitamin C lies within one mm of the skin's surface. And most of the fragrance cells are in the skin, so only have a tasteless fruit by peeling it.

The vitamin content decreases gradually towards the centre of the fruit. The skin also contains five times more vitamin A than the flesh.

Red apple skins are particularly rich in anthocyanins, which are antioxidants that may protect against several types of cancer, in particular prostate cancer. Yellow apple skins contain carotenoids like beta-carotene, which help maintain healthy eyes, combat cancers and protect against heart disease. And green apple skins are rich in lutein, which can help reduce the risk of cataracts and birth defects and also protect against cancers.

Add to the nutritive value of Apple. Dip slices in heart-healthy peanut butter. The protein-carbohydrate mix forms a perfect post-workout snack.

APRICOT

Botanical Name: *Prunus armeniaca*
Indian Name: *Khubāni, Zardālu*

Apricot is an important fruit belonging to the sub-acid class. It is somewhat acid in its raw state but this acidity decreases and the sugar content increases as it ripens. The fruit is a nutritious, tonic food which enjoys world-wide popularity.

Yellowish in colour, apricot is a stone fruit with a nut inside. It is round or oblong in shape. Somewhat similar to peach, but considerably smaller. Only the fruit which ripens on the tree develops true flavour and is much like that of the peach.

Origin and Distribution: Apricot is believed to have originated in China. It has also been grown in India and Tibet from time immemorial. The Hunzas, who live in the Himalayan mountains of northern Pakistan and known for their vitality and longevity, have cultivated and valued this fruit for its health for over 1,500 years. It was regarded as a food medicine by Greek physicians, while the Romans dedicated it to Venus, the goddess of love. In the Middle East, apricots are popular for their taste as well as for their perfume.

Food Value: Fresh apricots are rich in natural sugars, vitamin A and calcium. They are a good source of the vitamins B-complex, riboflavin, niacin and vitamin C. The nut of the apricot is rich in protein and fat and is considered as valuable as any other nut. It contains 40 to 45 per cent of an oil which is practically identical to almond oil in its physical as well as chemical properties.

Natural Benefits and Curative Properties

Throughout centuries, the fruit, its kernels and the oil and flowers been used in medicine. In China, a famous medicine known as 'Apricot Gold', was made from the kernels of trees which grew in select regions. This medicine was reputed for its powers to prolong life. The Chinese also believed that apricots reacted sympathetically

Fresh Apricot*

Food Value		Minerals and Vitamins	
Moisture	85.3%	Calcium	20 mg
Protein	1.0%	Phosphorus	25 mg
Fat	0.3%	Iron	2.2 mg
Minerals	0.7%	Vitamin C	6 mg
Fibre	1.0%	Small amounts of	
Carbohydrates	11.6%	Vitamin B Complex	
	100%		

Calorific Value - 53

Dried Apricot*

Food Value		Minerals and Vitamins	
Moisture	19.4%	Calcium	110 mg
Protein	1.6%	Phosphorus	70 mg
Fat	0.7%	Iron	4.6 mg
Minerals	2.8%	Vitamin C	2 mg
Fibre	2.1%	Small amounts of	
Carbohydrates	73.4%	Vitamin B Complex	
	100%		

**Values per 100 gms edible portion | Calorific Value - 306*

to women's ailments. The apricot flowers formed a common ingredient in their cosmetics.

The kernels, which yield an oil similar to almond oil, have been widely used for their sedative, antispasmodic (that give relief to inflammed muscles) and demulcent properties. They are also useful in the healing wounds, in expelling worms and as a general tonic.

Constipation

Due to its cellulose and pectin content the fruit is highly valued as a gentle laxative and is beneficial in treating constipation. The cellulose acts as a roughage and the pectin absorbs and retains water, thereby increasing bulk of faeces and stimulating a smooth bowel movement. Patients suffering from chronic constipation can greatly benefit by regular use of apricots. Generally six to eight apricots per day will produce the desired result.

Indigestion

Apricots have an alkaline reaction in the body. If taken before a meal they aid digestion. Marmalade made from organically grown fruit is also valuable in the treatment of nervous indigestion.

Anaemia

With its high iron content apricot is an excellent remedy for anaemia. A small but essential amount of copper in appricot is of great help. According to Dr. Whipple and Dr. Robschiet Robbins, production of haemoglobin can be increased with liberal use of apricots.[1]

Fevers

Fresh juice of apricots mixed with glucose or honey is a cooling drink during fevers. It quenches thirst and eliminates the waste products from the body. It tones up the eyes, stomach, liver, heart and nerves by supplying vitamins and minerals.

Skin Diseases

Fresh juice of apricot leaves is useful in skin diseases. It can be applied with beneficial results in scabies, eczema, sun-burn and itching of the skin due to cold exposure.

Uses

Apricot in its fresh form is mostly used as a dessert fruit. However, it is also used in its dried form. It is also made into jams, jelly, marmalades and preserves. Apricots canned in sugar are fairly popular. The nut of the apricot is extensively used in confectionary.

AVOCADO

Botanical Name: *Persea americana*
Indian Name: *Kulu Nāspāti or Mākhanphal*

Avocado is a large fleshy pear-shaped berry. It has a single large seed surrounded by buttery pulp and a hard skin. It is yellowish-green to maroon and purple in colour. The avocado tree is evergreen. It is shallow-rooted and there are no

1. Fairfax T. Proudfit, *Nutrition and Diet Therapy*, p. 251. Macmillan and Co., New York, 1934

visible root hairs. It has spirally-arranged leaves, variable in shape and size, and fragrant yellowish flowers.

Origin and Distribution: Avocado originated in the Central Americas. Early Spanish explorers recorded its cultivation from Mexico to Peru. It was taken to southern Spain in 1601. The fruit was introduced in Mauritius in 1780 and spread in Asia mostly in the mid-19th century. Avocados are now grown in most tropical and subtropical countries including South Africa and Australia.

Food Value: Avocado contains more fat than any other fruit except the olive. Its fat is of the highest quality, wholly free from the unpleasant butyric acid with which many fats are contaminated. It contains sufficient vitamin A to maintain high resistance against bacterial infection, a quality possessed only a few vegetable fats.

Avocado*

Food Value		**Minerals and Vitamins**	
Moisture	73.6%	Calcium	10 mg
Protein	1.7%	Phosphorus	80 mg
Fat	22.8%	Iron	0.7 mg
Minerals	1.1%	Vitamin A	290 IU**
Carbohydrates	0.8%	Sufficient amounts of Vit E & small amount of Vit C & Vit B Complex	
	100%		

**Values per 100 gms edible portion | Calorific Value - 215 | **Int'l Unit*

The protein of avocado is of the finest quality and much superior to protein of bread and other cereal foods. Its composition is almost identical with that of milk. In fact, the pulp of the fruit is free from fibre to such an extent that with water it forms a fine emulsion closely resembling milk in consistency and appearance. With the exception of an excess fat and lack of vitamin C, it can serve as a very satisfactory substitute for dairy milk. Prepared thus, avocado may be given safely to young infants and to invalids.

Natural Benefits and Curative Properties

For purity, wholesomeness, digestibility and adaptation to human needs avocado has few rivals.

Digestive System Disorders

Avocado is an excellent food remedy in acute digestive disorders. Its blandness is comforting to the hypersensitive surfaces of the stomach and duodenum, and its abundant vitamins reanimate the inflamed and crippled cells. For centuries physicians in China have prescribed its juice for colic and chills in the stomach. The Japanese employ the same remedy to treat ulceration of the intestines.

Avocado is an efficient aid in changing the intestinal flora to combat auto-intoxication, colitis and biliousness. In cases of hyperacidity avocado and well ripened papaya should be the staple diet. These are two most appropriate foods in cases of duodenitis and duodenal ulcer; they are bland, soothing to the sensitive membrane and pass quickly into the intestine.

Bad Breath

Avocado is far superior to any mouth wash or other remedies for bad breath. It effectively removes intestinal putrefactions which is the real cause of a coated tongue and bad breath.

Bright's Disease

In cases of Bright's disease avocado is especially useful as a staple food because of its small protein content.

Psoriasis

The oil of avocado is beneficial in treating psoriasis. It should be applied gently to the affected parts. It helps in taking the scales off.

Beauty Aid

Avocado oil is widely employed in preparing cosmetics. These include creams, cleansers and moisturizers to prevent the ageing effect of dehydration, skin foods, bath oils, shampoos which act as a scalp conditioner and revitalize dull hair.

Precautions: As avocados become sour when cooked and cannot successfully survive freezing, they should be eaten raw and as fresh as possible. If they have to be kept for a short period they should be stored at room temperature and not in a refrigerator.

BAEL FRUIT

Botanical Name: *Aegle marmelos*
Indian Name: *Bel, Siriphal*

Bael occupies an important place among the indigenous fruits of India. It is a woody and smooth fruit 5 to 15 cm in diameter, with numerous seeds, which are embedded in a thick aromatic pulp. The flesh is either eaten fresh or dried.

Origin and Distribution: History of bael tree can be traced to the Vedic period, 2000 BC - 800 BC. The fruit is mentioned in *Yajur Veda* and abounds in the vicinity of temples. It is held sacred by the Hindus and the leaves of the tree are traditionally used as a holy offering to Lord Shiva, who is said to live under bael tree.

Bael fruit is grown throughout India, and the entire Indian sub-continent; Thailand and most south-east Asian countries.

Food Value: An analysis of bael fruit shows that it is rich in mineral and vitamin content. *Sherbet* made of this fruit is rich in important nutrients and health improving ingredients. The *sherbet* should be thick and syrupy enough to be taken with a spoon and should be thoroughly masticated. If taken hurriedly, it may produce heaviness in the stomach. Excessive intake of bael fruit can also produce a sensation of heaviness in the stomach and gastric discomfort.

Natural Benefits and Curative Properties

The medicinal properties of bael have been described in the ancient Sanskrit medical treatise, *Charaka Samhita*. All parts of the tree, its

Bael*

Food Value		Minerals and Vitamins	
Moisture	61.5%	Calcium	85 mg
Protein	1.8%	Phosphorus	50 mg
Fat	0.3%	Iron	0.6 mg
Minerals	1.7%	Vitamin C	8 mg
Fibre	2.9%	Small amounts of	
Carbohydrates	31.8%	Vitamin B Complex	
	100%		

**Values per 100 gms edible portion | Calorific Value - 137*

stem, bark, root, leaves and the fruit at all stages of maturity have medicinal virtues and are used in the traditional medicine.

The ripe fruit is aromatic, an astringent, a coolant and a laxative. The unripe or half-ripe fruit acts as an astringent, improves appetite and is antiscorbutic, i.e. helps fight scurvy due to vitamin C deficiency.

Constipation

Ripe bael fruit is regarded as a good natural laxative. It cleans and tones the intestines. Its regular use for two or three months helps evacuate even the old accumulated faecal matter. For best results, it should be taken as *sherbet* prepared from the pulp of the ripe fruit. After breaking the shell, the seeds are removed, contents spooned out and passed through a sieve. Milk and little sugar may be added to make it more palatable. The pulp of the ripe fruit, about 60 gms, taken with a spoon without any addition should suffice for an adult.

> No disease that can be treated
> with diet should be treated
> with any other means.
> Ryan Frimmel

Diarrhoea and Dysentery

The unripe or half ripe fruit is perhaps the most effective remedy for chronic diarrhoea and dysentery when there is no fever. Best results are obtained using dried bael or its powder. The bael fruit, when still green, is sliced and dried in the sun. The dried slices are powdered and preserved in air-tight bottles. The unripe bael can be baked and taken with jaggery or brown sugar.

The fruit appears to have little effect in acute dysentery when only some blood and mucus pass out. The powdered drug is recommended in this condition. Its beneficial effect is, however, most evident when the condition is sub-acute or chronic. After the use of the fruit in these conditions, blood gradually disappears and the stool assumes a more feculent and solid form. The mucus also disappears with regular use for some time. It is also a valuable remedy for chronic dysentery condition characterised by alternate diarrhoea and constipation.[1]

Peptic Ulcer

An infusion of bael leaves is regarded as an effective remedy for peptic ulcer. The leaves are soaked overnight in water, the water strained and taken in the morning. Both pain and discomfort are relieved with continued treatment for a few weeks. Bael leaves are rich in tannins which reduce inflammation and help healing of ulcers. Also bael fruit taken as a beverage has multiple healing properties on account of its mucilage, i.e. sticky or viscous content. This substance forms a coating on the stomach mucosa and thus helps in the healing of ulcers.

Respiratory Affections

A medicated oil prepared from bael leaves gives relief from recurrent colds and respiratory affections. The juice extracted from bael leaves is mixed with equal quantity of sesame oil and thoroughly heated. A few seeds of black pepper and half a teaspoonful of black cumin are added to the hot oil. It is then removed from the fire and stored for use. A teaspoonful of this oil massaged regularly into the scalp before a head bath builds resistance against colds and coughs.

A common practice in south India is to give the juice of bael leaves to bring relief from wheezing and respiratory spasm. The leaf juice, mixed in warm water and a little pepper, is given as a drink.

---

1. Col. Chopra, *Indigenous Drugs of India*, p. 269, Academic Publishers. Calcutta. 1982

BANANA

Botanical Name: *Musa paradisiaca*
Indian Name: *Kelā*

Banana is one of the oldest and perhaps the best known fruit of the world. It is delicious, seedless and available in all seasons at a reasonable price. Its thick covering provides an excellent protection against bacteria and contamination. The mature fruit may be greenish, yellow or reddish in colour.

Origin and Distribution: Original home of banana is believed to be India and Malaya (now Malaysia). Greek and Arab writers referred to it as a wonder fruit of India. The fruit as well as its plant is considered to be very auspicious in religious and social ceremonies in India. The Malayan soldiers probably took it to Madagascar about the fifth century AD and from there it spread to mainland Africa and other parts of the world. In India the important banana-producing areas are South India, West India and East India.

Food Value: Banana is a rare combination of energy value, tissue-building elements, protein, vitamins and minerals. Being richer in solids and lower in water content than any other fresh fruit it is a good source of calories. A large banana supplies more than 100 calories. It contains large amounts of easily assimilable sugar, making it a good source of quick energy and recovery from fatigue.

In combination with milk, banana constitutes almost a complete balanced diet. It contains a high grade protein, which includes three of the essential amino acids. Banana and milk supplement each other in ideally and provide all the needed nutrients to the body.

Natural Benefits and Curative Properties

In traditional Indian and Persian medicine this golden fruit is regarded as nature's secret of perpetual youth. It helps promote retention of calcium, phosphorus and nitrogen — all of which work to build sound and regenerated tissues. Banana also contains invert sugar, which is an aid to youthful growth and metabolism.

Banana*

Food Value		Minerals and Vitamins	
Moisture	70.1%	Calcium	17 mg
Protein	1.2%	Phosphorus	36 mg
Fat	0.3%	Iron	0.9 mg
Minerals	0.8%	Vitamin C	7 mg
Fibre	0.4%	Small amounts of	
Carbohydrates	27.2%	Vitamin B Complex	
	100%		

**Values per 100 gms edible portion | Calorific Value - 116*

Intestinal Disorder

Because of its soft texture and blandness, banana is used as a dietary food in intestinal disorders. It is said to contain an unidentified compound perhaps jokingly called, 'vitamin U' (against ulcer). It is the only raw fruit which can be eaten without distress in chronic ulcer. It neutralises over-acidity of gastric juices and reduces irritation of the ulcer by coating the stomach lining.

Being bland, smooth, easily-digestible and slightly laxative, ripe bananas are highly beneficial in the treatment of ulcerative colitis. They relieve acute symptoms and promote the healing process.

Constipation and Diarrhoea

Bananas are of great value both in constipation and diarrhoea as they normalise colonic functions in the large intestine to absorb large amounts of water for proper bowel moments. Their usefulness is due to their being rich in pectin, which is water-absorbent and this gives them a bulk producing ability. They also possess the ability to change the bacteria in the intestines — from the harmful type of bacilli to the beneficial acidophyllus bacilli.

Dysentery

Mashed banana with a little salt added is a valuable remedy for dysentery. According to Dr. Kirticar, a combination of ripe plantain, tamarind and common salt is most effective in this disease. He claims to have cured several cases of both acute and chronic dysentery with this treatment.[1] Ripe bananas are also very useful in

1. Lt. Col. Kirticar and Major R.D. Basu, *Indian Medical Plants* pp. 1268, Allahabad, 1918.

dysentery of children, but they should be thoroughly mashed and beaten to cream before being given to children.

Arthritis and Gout

Bananas are useful in the treatment of arthritis and gout. A diet consisting of bananas for three or four days is advised in these conditions. The patient can be given eight or nine bananas daily during this period and nothing else.

Anaemia

Being high in iron content, bananas are beneficial in treating anaemia. They stimulate the production of haemoglobin.

Allergies

The fruit is very useful for those who are allergic to other foods and suffer from skin rashes, digestive disorders or asthma. Unlike other protein foods, many of which contain an amino-acid which allergic persons cannot tolerate, bananas contain only benign amino-acids which in most cases are not allergic. The fruit, however, may cause allergic reactions in some highly sensitive persons.

Kidney Disorders

With their low protein and salt content and high carbohydrate content bananas are valuable in kidney disorders. They are useful in uraemia, a toxic condition of the blood due to kidney congestion and dysfunction. In such cases, a diet of bananas should only be taken for three to four days, consuming eight to nine bananas a day. This diet is suitable for all kidney troubles, including nephritis.

Tuberculosis

Bananas are considered useful in the treatment of tuberculosis. According to Dr. J. Montelvz of Brazil, the juice of the plantain or cooked ordinary bananas works miracles in curing tuberculosis. With this treatment he claims to have cured patients in advanced stage of tuberculosis accompanied with frequent cough, abundant expectoration or phlegm and high fever in two months.[1]

---

1. Dr. S.J. Singh, *Food Remedies*, pp. 42, Nature Cure Council of Medical Research, Lucknow, 1982.

Urinary Disorders

Juice from banana stem is a well-known remedy for urinary disorders. It improves the functional efficiency of kidney and liver thereby alleviating their diseased condition and the patient discomfort. It clears the abdominal region of toxins and helps to eliminate them in the form of urine. It has also been found to be helpful in the treatment of kidney stones, gall bladder stones, and prostate. Whenever possible it is advisable to mix this juice with the juice of ash pumpkin.

Over-weight/Obesiy/Slimming

Bananas are suitable for overweight people as they contain practically no sodium. A diet consisting of bananas and skimmed milk is considered an effective remedy for weight reduction. Daily diet is restricted to six bananas and four glasses of skimmed milk or buttermilk (made from skimmed milk) for a period of 10 to 15 days. Thereafter green vegetables may be gradually introduced, reducing the intake of bananas from six to four. This regimen can be continued till desired results are achieved.

Menstrual Disorders

Cooked banana flower eaten with curd is considered an effective medicine for menstrual disorders like painful menstruation and excessive bleeding. Banana flower helps increase progesterone hormone which reduces the bleeding.[1]

Burns and Wounds

A plaster prepared by beating a ripe banana into a fine paste and applied over burns and wounds and supported by a cloth bandage gives immediate relief. The young tender leaves of banana tree form a cool dressing for inflammations and blisters.

Uses

Ripe bananas are chiefly eaten as a dessert or a breakfast fruit. They are also used in salads with other fruits. Unripe fruits are cooked.

---

1. Dr. Aman, *Medical Secrets of Your Foods*, pp. 190, Indo-American Hospital, Mysore, 1985.

Banana chips are made from fully mature unripe fruits. The flour prepared from the dried unripe bananas is three times richer in minerals than the wheat flour. It is also more digestible than cereal starches and an ideal food for infants and invalids.

Precautions: Banana, taken as a table fruit, must be ripe else it may be difficult to digest. Raw bananas contain 20 to 25 per cent starch which during the process of ripening is almost wholly converted with assimilable sugar.

Bananas should never be kept in a refrigerator; low temperature prevents their ripening. The fruit should not be taken by those suffering from kidney failure because of its high potassium content.

DATE

Botanical Name: *Phoenix dactylifera*
Indian Name: *Khajur*

Date is one of the most nourishing fruits. It was once famous as the bread of the Sahara but its use is now universal. It is included in the categories of both dry and fresh fruit. Date is a cylindrical fruit of yellow to reddish brown colour. It has a fleshy pericarp surrounding a single seed containing 60 to 70 per cent sugar. The palm tree-ripe fresh date is delicious. It however ferments very rapidly and is, therefore, dried in the sun. The fruit looses about 35 per cent of its weight in the process of drying.

Origin and Distribution: Date has been held in high esteem from the ancient times and is one of the earliest cultivated fruits. There are numerous references to the palm and its fruit in the Bible. Prophet Mohammed believed that the first date palm was made from the tempered dust which remained after the formation of Adam.

The original home of date is believed to be the Persian Gulf area or Mesopotamia. It is now a standard crop widely grown in Saudi Arabia, Egypt, Iran, Iraq, Spain, China and U.S.A.

Food Value: The date is of high nutritional value. It provides natural sugar in the form of glucose and fructose which is immediately absorbed in the body and is therefore infinitely superior to cane-sugar. Dates are usually taken raw or with milk, and this makes them highly nutritious in most respects. Taking dates with curdled milk is common. In Sahara, the rich take it after removing the seed and filling the cavity with butter. It is a scientific way of taking fat. The seeds of the fruit, roasted and ground into powder makes a coffee like beverage, called 'date coffee'. The date palm yields a sweet juice of high food value. It can be taken fresh or made into a tasty country sugar. The juice can also be fermented and made into alcohol.

Date*

Food Value		**Minerals and Vitamins**	
Moisture	15.3%	Calcium	120 mg
Protein	2.5%	Phosphorus	50 mg
Fat	0.4%	Iron	7.3 mg
Minerals	2.1%	Vitamin C	3 mg
Fibre	3.9%	Small amounts of	
Carbohydrates	75.8%	Vitamin B Complex	
	100%		

**Values per 100 gms edible portion | Calorific Value - 317*

Natural Benefits and Curative Properties

Dates are valuable as medicine for their tonic effect. Being easily digested, they are very useful for supplying energy and repairing waste. Milk in which clean and fresh dates have been boiled makes a very nourishing and restorative drink for children and adults alike, especially during convalescence.

Intestinal Health

The nicotinic content in dates is an excellent remedy for intestinal disturbances. According to Metchnikoff, the great Russian scientist, liberal use of dates keeps the growth of pathological organisms in check and helps friendly bacteria in the intestines.[1]

1. K.R.Mukherjee, *Protective Foods in Health and Disease,* pp 53, Prakritick Chikitsalaya, Culcatta, 4th edition, 1983.

Constipation

Date is a laxative food. The roughage provided by it stimulates sluggish bowels thus helping to treat constipation. For maximum laxative effect dates are best immersed in water at night and taken after making them into a fine syrup the next morning.

Intoxication

Dates are an excellent remedy for alcoholic intoxication. Drinking water in which fresh dates have been soaked brings quick relief.

Weak Heart

Dates are an effective remedy for a weak heart. Dates soaked overnight in water and crushed after removing the seeds in the same water the next morning should be taken at least twice a week in this condition. This helps to strengthen the heart.

Sexual Debility

A handful of dates soaked in fresh goat's milk overnight should be ground in the same milk the next morning. With a pinch of cardamom powder and honey mixed it makes for a very useful tonic for improving sex stamina and sterility caused by functional disorders.[1]

Children's Diseases

According to Dr. Aman, a date tied to the wrist of a baby and allowed to be sucked during teething time hardens the gums and also prevents complaints like fretfulness and diarrhoea. A teaspoonful of paste of a date prepared with honey and given thrice a day is an effective medicine for diarrhoea and dysentery during teething[2] is another good remedy.

Precautions: The sticky surface of the fruit attracts dust and impurities. It is, therefore, advisable to buy the best varieties, well packed, and to wash them thoroughly before use.

---

1. Dr. Aman, *Medicinal Secrets of Your Food*, pp 201, Indo American Hospital, Mysore, 1985.
2. Ibid., p. 202.

FIG

Botanical Name: *Ficus carica*
Indian Name: *Anjeer*

Fig occupies a high position among fruits. This delicious pear-shaped health promoting fruit is soft, sweet and pulpy. It is a hollow fruit, with sugary pulp and a large number of golden coloured small seeds sticking to the wall of the cavity. Being highly perishable, it is mostly sold in its dry form. The dry fig has a high nutritive value.

Origin and Distribution: The fig is a native of Asia Minor and spread early to the Mediterranean region. It was grown in Egypt around 4,000 BC. The main areas of fig cultivation in India are in Maharashtra, Karnataka, Uttar Pradesh and parts of Gujarat.

Food Value: Fresh fig consists of good amount of moisture and small amounts of protein, fat and carbohydrate. The most important food element of a fig is sugar which forms 51 to 74 per cent of the whole fruit. It can be taken by itself or in combination with other foodstuffs to enrich their food value. When taken with white flour, it removes much of its constipating effect. It combines very well with milk. Figs are often used in cakes, jams and puddings.

Natural Benefits and Curative Properties

Many medicinal virtues have been ascribed to the fig. It is considered a restorative food which helps in quick recovery after prolonged illness. It removes physical and mental exertion and restores vigour and strength. It is an excellent tonic for weak individuals who suffer cracked lips, tongue and mouth.

Constipation

Taken fresh or dried fig is a dependable laxative due to its large cellulose content and its tough skin. The tiny seeds in the fruit stimulate peristaltic or wave like movements of intestines which facilitates easy evacuation and keeps the alimentary canal clean.

Fig* (Fresh)

Food Value		Minerals and Vitamins	
Moisture	88.1%	Calcium	35 mg
Protein	1.3%	Phosphorus	22 mg
Fat	0.2%	Iron	0.6 mg
Minerals	7.6%	Vitamin A	80 IU**
Fibre	2.2%	Vitamin C	2 mg
Carbohydrates	0.6%	Small amounts of	
	100%	Vitamin B Complex	

*Calorific Value - 80 | **Int'l Unit*

Fig* (Dry)

Food Value		Minerals and Vitamins	
Moisture	23.0%	Calcium	126 mg
Protein	4.3%	Phosphorus	77 mg
Fat	1.3%	Iron	3 mg
Minerals	63.4%	Vitamin A	80 IU**
Fibre	5.6%	Small amounts of	
Carbohydrates	2.4%	Vitamin B Complex	
	100%		

**Values per 100 gms edible portion | Calorific Value - 274 | **Int'l Unit*

Piles

Owing to its laxative property, fig is an excellent remedy for piles. After a thorough cleaning with hot water two or three dried figs should be soaked in cold water overnight and taken the next morning and evening. This eliminates straining to pass stool and prevents protrusion of the anus. Piles can be cured with regular use of figs in this manner for three or four weeks.

Asthma

Figs are considered beneficial in treating phlegmatic asthma and cough. It helps by draining the phlegm.

Sexual Weakness

Figs can be beneficially used in treating sexual debility. They can be supplemented by other dry fruits like almonds and dry dates along with butter. Their use has proved effective in such cases.

Corns

The milky juice of green figs helps to soften corns of long duration. The milk has a mild necrotic action.

Precautions: Figs should always be washed thoroughly before use. The skin of the dry fruit being tough, the soaked fig is easy to digest. It is essential to take the water along with the fruit as much of the nutrients come out into the water.

GRAPES

Botanical Name: *Vitis vinifera*
Indian Name: *Angoor*

Grapes are nature's precious gift to man. They are amongst the most valuable of fruits — delicious, highly nutritious and easily digestible.

Grapes are a form of berry. There are innumerable varieties differing in size, shape, colour, aroma and taste. They grow in various colours such as green, black, red and blue.

Origin and Distribution: Grapes are one of the earliest fruit vines cultivated. The 8,000 year old monuments of Egypt contain carvings of grapes on stone. Grapes are believed to be indigenous to Caucasia region. From here this fruit spread to Western Asia, Southern Europe, Algeria, Morocco and India. The main centres of grape cultivation in India are in Tamil Nadu, Maharashtra, Telangana, Himachal, Punjab and Uttar Pradesh.

Food Value: Grapes are highly valued for their rich content of sugar which is formed almost entirely of glucose. The quantity of glucose in grapes varies from 15 to 25 per cent depending upon the variety. The glucose is a pre-digested food and absorbed in the body soon after its consumption. It supplies heat and energy to the body within a short time.

Natural Benefits and Curative Properties

The therapeutic value of grapes is closely linked to its pure glucose. Studies have indicated that the production of energy essential for proper functioning of the heart and organs of high physiological

Grapes*

Food Value		Minerals and Vitamins	
Moisture	92.0%	Calcium	20 mg
Protein	0.7%	Phosphorus	20 mg
Fat	0.1%	Iron	0.2 mg
Minerals	0.2%	Vitamin C	31 mg
Carbohydrates	7.0%	Small amounts of Vit B Complex, Vitamin A and P	
	100%		

**Values per 100 gms edible portion | Calorific Value - 32*

importance depends on metabolism of glucose. By virtue of their easy assimilation, grapes have a restorative effect. They are highly valued in strengthening weak digestion, overcoming general debility and fever.

'Grape cure' is perhaps the best of the various fruit cures. It consists of eating a daily diet exclusively of grapes. As far back as 1556, books on this wonderful method of natural treatment had been published in Europe. Over a hundred years ago, Dr. Lambe, a pioneer dietitian, treated cancer in England with grapes. Germany seems to have been the centre of this natural healing cult.

Grape diet is recommended by Prof. Dr. Herman Rieder and Dr. Martin Zeller, both of Munchen, Germany. For a complete cure these doctors prescribe the juice extracted from fresh grapes to be taken five times a day. The treatment lasts from four to six weeks and the best time for this diet are the months of September and October. In some cases large quantities of juice are administered — from 1 to 6.5 kg of pressed grapes being used daily.[1]

Constipation

The combination of cellulose, sugar and organic acid in the grapes makes them an effective laxative food, highly valuable in relieving constipation. However its action is not limited in clearing the bowels only. It tones up the stomach and intestines and relieves the most chronic cases of constipation. One should take atleast 350 gms of grapes daily to achieve the desired results. When fresh grapes are not available, raisins soaked in water can be used.

1. Johanna Brandt, *The Grape Cure*, pp. 147-148, Ehret Literature Publising Co., California.

Dyspepsia

Grapes constitute a light food which cures indigestion and stomach irritation in a short time and relieves heat.

Asthma

According to Dr. Oldfield, grapes and their juices are beneficial in the treatment of asthma. He thinks that the patient can recover early if he is kept in a garden of grapes.[1]

Heart Disease

Grapes are highly beneficial in the treatment of heart disease. They tone up the heart and are effective in cardiac pain and palpitation of the heart. The disease can be rapidly controlled with an exclusive grape diet for few days. Grape juice is said to be valuable when one is suffering from a heart attack. This helps avert serious consequences by reducing pain and palpitation.

Migraine

Juice of ripe grapes is an effective home remedy for migraine. It is said that King Jamshed, who was very fond of grapes, once stored juice of grapes well packed in bottles and made it public that the bottles contained strong poison so as to prevent others from taking it. It so happened that the wife of the king was struck with migraine and having obtained no relief from any treatment, decided to end her life by taking this so called 'poison'. She took it several times in small doses and contrary to her expectations, it gave her great relief instead of killing her.[2]

Kidney Troubles

Grapes have an exceptional diuretic value on account of their being high in water and potassium content. Its value in kidney troubles is enhanced by low content of albumin and sodium chloride. It is an excellent food remedy in acute and chronic nephritis and in cases of kidney and bladder stones.

---

1. Kvj. Ganpati Singh Verma, *Miracles of Fruits*, pp. 23, The Rasayan Pharmacy, New Delhi, 9th Edition 1978.
2. Ibid p. 5

Liver Disorders

Grapes activate the liver or hepatic functions to stimulate glycogenic functions and bile secretion. They are thus highly beneficial in the treatment of liver disorders.

Children's Diseases

Grape juice is an excellent blood-builder. It is an effective household remedy and can be preserved in bottles. It is valuable to children in treating constipation and also in preventing convulsions due to constipation. The juice is an effective food remedy for infants during teething trouble.

External Sores

Grape poultices have been found effective in cases of growths an open sore. A poultice is prepared by crushing grapes and spreading them between layers of cheese cloth or muslin. The poultice is placed over the affected parts and covered with a dry cloth and renewed frequently. It absorbs much of the toxins.[1]

Pyorrhoea

The organic acids of the grapes are strongly antiseptic and their effect on the gums is very effective. According to Johanna Brandt, 'Every tooth may be loose in its socket and pus may be pouring from the gums, but after a few weeks on the exclusive grape diet it will be found that the teeth are firmly set in the jaw and that every trace of pyorrhoea poisoning has disappeared'.

Alcoholism

Grapes are highly beneficial in treating alcoholism and can be an exclusive diet in treating alcoholism.

Precautions: Grapes have a poor keeping quality; they undergo quick putrefaction. They should be used soon after purchase or preserved in cold storage. Only fully ripe grapes should be purchased.

---

1. Johanna Brandt, *The Grape Cure*, pp. 89, Ehret Literature Publishing Co., California.

GRAPEFRUIT

Botanical Name: *Citrus paradisi*
Indian Name: *Chakotrā*

Grapefruit occupies a high place among citrus fruits because of its flavour, appetising properties and refreshing qualities. It varies in colour and may have a pale yellow or pinkish flesh. The rind is usually one to one and a half cms thick.

Origin and Distribution: Grapefruit is indigenous to Indo-China, Thailand and Malaya region. It spread to other tropical countries from these lands and is now grown in West Indies, Israel, Brazil, South Africa, Australia, New Zealand, U.S.A. and India.

Food Value: The fruit is nutritive and refrigerant, and possesses much the same properties as the orange, lemon and lime. The seedless variety is the best; it often contains greater amount of sugar, calcium and phosphorus. Grapefruit is often used as table salad with other fruit and vegetables. It is sometimes cut into half, the seeds and the hard pith removed and the cavity sprinkled with sugar over the surface, left for an hour in a covered plate and then taken.

Grapefruit*

Food Value		**Minerals and Vitamins**	
Moisture	92.0%	Calcium	20 mg
Protein	0.7%	Phosphorus	20 mg
Fat	0.1%	Iron	0.2 mg
Minerals	0.2%	Vitamin C	31 mg
Carbohydrates	7.0%	Small amounts of Vit B Complex,	
	100%	A and P (Flavonoids)	

**Values per 100 gms edible portion | Calorific Value - 32*

Natural Benefits and Curative Properties

Grapefruit is an excellent appetiser. It promotes salivary and gastric digestion. It is an important health builder and a tonic.

Acidity

Inspite of its often sharp, sub-acid taste, fresh grapefruit has an alkaline reaction after digestion. The citric acid of the fruit is oxidized in the human system and hence the effect is to increase alkalinity of the body. The grapefruit juice is beneficial in preventing, controlling and treating acidity and other problems caused by excess acid in the system.

Digestive Disorders

The pulp of grapefruit supplies healthy bulk to aid bowel action. It is beneficial in maintaining health of the intestines and is regarded as a food which prevents dysentery, diarrhoea, enteritis, typhus and other infective diseases of the digestive tract.

Diabetes

According to Dr. Joe Shelby Riley, a well-known nutrition expert, 'Grapefruit is a splendid food for a diabetic patient. If grapefruits were eaten more liberally, there would be much less diabetes. Those with a tendency towards high sugar and want to prevent it, can take three a day and decrease starches and fats. Mostly fruits, vegetables and juices are advised. In two weeks sugar will be restored to normal level without need of insulin. In those on insulin, it takes longer.'[1]

Influenza

Juice of grapefruit is an excellent remedy for influenza. It helps to reduce acidity and its bitter properties due to the presence of a substance called 'maringin', which tones up the system and the digestive tract.

Fever

Grapefruit juice is an excellent diet in all kinds of fevers. It quenches thirst and removes the burning sensation produced by fever. Juice should be taken diluted with water.

Malaria

The fruit contains a natural 'quinine' and is valuable in treating malaria. This 'quinine' is also beneficial in feverish colds. It can be extracted by boiling a quarter of a grapefruit and straining the pulp.[2]

---

1. Dr. S.J. Singh, *Food Remedies*, pp. 103, Nature Cure Council of Medical Research, Lucknow, 1982.
2. Helen Jeans, *About Tropical Fruits*, pp. 32, Thorsons Publishers Limited, London 1972.

Fatigue
A glass of grapefruit and lemon juice in equal parts is an excellent way overcome fatigue and tiredness after a hard day's work.

Scanty Urination
Juice of grapefruit is extremely rich in vitamin C and potassium. It can, therefore, be beneficially used as a medicine in scanty urination caused by liver, kidney and heart disorders.

INDIAN GOOSEBERRY

Botanical Name: *Emblica officinalis*
Indian Name: *Amlā*

Indian gooseberry is a wonderful fruit and perhaps one of the most precious gifts of nature. It is the richest known natural source of vitamin C. This vitamin is readily assimilated by the body and contributes greatly towards health and longevity.

Indian gooseberry is globular, small, round, six-lobed fruit, thick and hard in consistency. It is light yellow in colour and about 1.25 cm to 2.5 cm in diameter.

Origin and Distribution: Indian gooseberry is indigenous to India. It has been used as a valuable ingredient various medicines in India and the Middle East from time immemorial. *Susrut*, the great Ayurvedic authority, considers it as the best of all acid fruits and one that is most useful in maintaing good health and recovering from disease. Like Ayurvedic physicians, Hakims of Unani medicine also use it frequently and regard it as a good medicine for heart and other problems. Due to its cool and astringent properties it is also used as an external application.

Indian gooseberry is grown as a commercial crop primarily in Uttar Pradesh. It also grows wild at the foot of the Himalayas and at elevation upto 1,500 metres in South India. The tree flowers in spring and fruit ripens in the winter.

Food Value: Indian gooseberry is valued chiefly for its high vitamin C content. The vitamin C value of *amla* increases further when juice is extracted from the fruit. The dehydrated berry provides 2428 to 3470 mg of vitamin C per 100 gms. Even when dried in the shade and turned into powder, it retains as much as 1780 to 2660 mg of Vitamin C.

The best way to take it with the least loss of vitamin C is to eat it raw with a little salt. The berry may also be used as a vegetable. It is often used in the form of pickles and marmalade. It can be preserved for a long periods when dried and turned into a powder.

Indian Gooseberry*

Food Value		Minerals and Vitamins	
Moisture	81.8%	Calcium	50 mg
Protein	0.5%	Phosphorus	20 mg
Fat	0.1%	Iron	1.2 mg
Minerals	0.5%	Vitamin C	600 mg
Fibre	3.4%	Small amounts of	
Carbohydrates	13.7%	Vitamin B Complex	
	100%		

**Values per 100 gms edible portion | Calorific Value - 48*

Natural Benefits and Curative Properties

The fresh fruit is light, laxative and diuretic. A tablespoonful each of fresh gooseberry juice mixed with honey forms a very valuable medicine for treating several ailments. If fresh fruit is not available, dry powder can be mixed with honey. Taken regularly every morning it promotes vigour within a few days.

Respiratory Disorders

This medicinal tonic is highly beneficial in treatment of respiratory disorders. It is especially valuable in tuberculosis of the lungs, asthma and bronchitis.

Diabetes

Indian gooseberry, with its high vitamin C content, is considered valuable in diabetes. A tablespoonful of its juice, mixed with a cup of fresh bitter gourd juice, taken daily for two months stimulates the islets of Lengerhans i.e. the isolated group of cells that secrete the hormone insulin. This reduces blood sugar in diabetes. Diet restrictions need to be strictly observed while taking this medicine. It also prevents diabetes related eye complications.[1]

Equal quantity of *amla* powder, *jamun* powder and bitter-gourd powder also make a very useful remedy for diabetics. A teaspoonful of this mixture once or twice a day is effective in checking the progress of the disease.

Heart Disease

Indian gooseberry is considered an effective remedy for heart disease. It tones up functioning of all organs and restores health and renews physical and mental energy.

Eye Disorders

Juice of Indian gooseberry mixed with honey is useful in preserving eyesight. It is also beneficial in treating conjunctivitis and glaucoma. It reduces intraocular tension. A cupful of this juice mixed with honey should be taken twice a day in such cases.

Rheumatism

One teaspoonful of powder of the dry fruit mixed with two teaspoonfuls of jaggery is recommended twice daily for a month in treating rheumatism.[2]

Scurvy

As an extremely rich source of vitamin C, Indian gooseberry is one of the best remedies for scurvy. Powder of dry gooseberry mixed with equal quantity of sugar should be taken in doses of one teaspoonful thrice daily with milk.

Diarrhoea and Dysentery

The dried fruit is valuable in diarrhoea and dysentery. A drink made from *amla* mixed with lemon juice and *misri* is highly beneficial in controlling acute bacillary dysentery. A tablespoonful of paste of leaves mixed with honey or butter-milk also makes an effective medicine.

---

1. Dr. Aman, *Medical Secrets of Your Food*, pp. 399, Indo American Hospital, Mysore, 1985.
2. Ibid., p. 400.

Premature Ageing

Indian gooseberry has revitalising effects. It contains a valuable element which helps to slow down ageing and also in maintaining strength in old age. It improves immunity against infection. It strengthens the heart, hair and different glands in the body. It is said that the great ancient sage Muni Chyawan rejuvenated himself in the seventh decade of his life and regained virility by using *amla.*

Hair Tonic

Indian gooseberry is an accepted traditional hair tonic for enriching hair growth and hair pigmentation. The fruit, cut into small pieces is dried, preferably in shade. These pieces are boiled in coconut oil till the solid matter becomes like charred dust. This darkish oil is excellent for preventing greying. The water in which dired *amla* pieces are soaked overnight also nourishes hair. This water should be used for the last rinse during hair wash.[1]

JAMUN FRUIT

Botanical Name: *Syzygium cumini or Eugenia jambolana*

Indian Name: *Jāmun*

Jamun is a well-known fruit. It has two varieties. The larger one is oval shaped and is commonly called as *Suva-jumun.* The smaller one is round and is commonly known as *kala-jamun.* The bigger variety is sweeter than the smaller one.

The fruit is a juicy berry with a single stone. It is black outside and violet inside; has a sourish-sweet pulp and greenish yellow seed.

Origin and Distribution: Jamun fruit is considered to be a native of India but is now found in all tropical regions and grows abundantly in the rainy season. It is found in most parts of India.

1. Dr. Girija Khanna, *Herbal Remedies*, pp. 127, Tarang Paperbacks, New Delhi, 1982.

Jamun Fruit*

Food Value		Minerals and Vitamins	
Moisture	83.7%	Calcium	15 mg
Protein	0.7%	Phosphorus	15 mg
Fat	0.3%	Iron	1.2 mg
Minerals	0.4%	Vitamin C	18 mg
Fibre	0.9%	Small amounts of	
Carbohydrates	14.0%	Vitamin B Complex	
	100%		

**Values per 100 gms edible portion | Calorific Value - 62*

Natural Benefits and Curative Properties

Diabetes

In traditional medicine jamun fruit is regarded as specific against diabetes because of its effect on the pancreas. The fruits, the seeds and its juice are all useful in treatment of this disease. The seeds contain a glucose 'jamboline' which is believed to check conversion of starch into sugar. The seeds are dried and powdered. This powder dissolved in water and given three or four times a day in doses of three grams. It reduces the sugar level in urine.

In Ayurveda, the inner bark of the jamun tree is also used in treating diabetes. The bark is dried and burnt producing a white coloured ash. This ash is pestled in the mortar, strained and bottled. The diabetic patient is given 65 mg of this ash with water on empty stomach in the mornings and 135 mg each an hour after meals, if the specific gravity of urine is 1.02 to 1.03. If the specific gravity ranges between 1.035 and 1.055, the ash should be given thrice daily in the quantity of about 2 gm at a time.[1]

Polyuria

The powder of the seeds is valuable in polyuria or production of excess urine. A dose of 1 gm in the morning and evening is advised.

Diarrhoea and Dysentery

Powder of the seed is an effective remedy for diarrhoea and dysentery. About 5 to 10 gm of this powder should be taken with

1. Kvj. Ganpati. Singh Verma, *Miracles of Indian Herbs*, pp. 61, Rasayan Pharmacy, 1982.

butter-milk in these conditions. An infusion of tender leaves which contain a high concentration of gallic and tannic acid is also given in diarrhoea and dysentery. This infusion, prepared from 30 or 60 gm of leaves, should be given twice or thrice daily. A decoction of the bark taken with honey is also useful.[1]

Piles

Jamun fruit is an effective remedy for bleeding piles. In season, the fruit should be taken with salt every morning for two or three months. This regimen should be continued life-long. This will effect radical cure and rid bleeding piles for life. Fresh jamun fruit taken with honey is also effective for bleeding piles.

Liver Disorders

Natural acids in the jamun fruit play an important role in secretion of digestive enzymes and stimulate liver function. *Charaka*, the well-known physician of the ancient India, used this fruit for treating enlarged liver.

Female sterility

An infusion of the fresh tender leaves of jamun fruit, taken with honey or butter-milk, is an effective remedy for sterility and miscarriage due to ovarian or endometrium functional disorder.

Precautions: Excessive use jamun fruit is bad for throat and chest. It may cause cough and accumulation of sputum in the lungs.

A must-eat rainy season fruit !

Jamun is rich in protein, fibre, antioxidants, calcium, iron, potassium, manganese, vitamin C and B_6 and several other nutrients. Clearly, it qualifies as a superfood that should be consumed on a regular basis. Still better, jamun is not very high in calorie count.

1. Dr. Aman, Medicinal Secrets of Your Food, pp. 223-224, Indo-American Hospital, Mysore, 1985.

LEMON

Botanical Name: *Citrus limon*
Indian Names: *Bara nimbu, Pahari nimbu*

Lemon is an important fruit of the citrus group and ranked high as health food. Sometimes it is mistaken for lime, but lime is smaller than lemon. Lemon is the bigger variety with rough, thin and loose rind. It is light yellow in colour with thick, rough skin and oval shape. When ripe it has pale yellow pulp, abundant juice and a small number of seeds.

Origin and Distribution: Lemon is indigenous to the north-west regions of India. It reached Europe in the 12th and 13th centuries. It is now widely grown in all tropical and subtropical countries, notably USA, Spain, Portugal, France, West Indies and New South Wales. In India, lemon is also cultivated in home gardens.

Food Value: Lemon is rich in multiple food ingredients, particularly citric acid. Different varieties contain this acid in proportions ranging from 3.71 to 8.40 per cent. It is mainly due to its citric acid and vitamin C content that lemon is widely used in medicines. Its juice is valued and also used as an accessory food to increases flavour of various dishes. It is often used in preparing salads and in preventing discolouration of sliced bananas and apple. It is widely used in the preparation of lemonades, squashes, jams, jellies and marmalades. Lemon juice has good keeping quality and can be preserved for a long time with precautions.

Natural Benefits and Curative Properties

The various parts of lemon used for medicinal purposes are rind of the ripe fruit, essential oil of the rind and expressed juice of the ripe fruit. A pale yellow volatile oil is derived either through distillation or by squeezing from fresh outer part of the pericarp of the fruit. Though bitter, the oil is highly valued in medicine as a flavouring agent, a carminative that relives flatulence, is used for treating gastric discomfort and improving appetite. Rind is also both a stomachic and a carminative.

Lemon*

Food Value		Minerals and Vitamins	
Moisture	85.0%	Calcium	70 mg
Protein	1.0%	Phosphorus	10 mg
Fat	0.9%	Iron	2.3 mg
Minerals	0.3%	Vitamin C	39 mg
Fibre	1.7%	Small amounts of	
Carbohydrates	11.1%	Vitamin B Complex	
	100%		

**Values per 100 gms edible portion | Calorific Value - 57*

The expressed and strained juice of a ripe lemon is valuable as an antiscorbutic and as a refrigerant. It destroys the toxins present in the body. This detoxifying property arises from its high potassium content. The germs of diphtheria, typhoid and other diseases are destroyed by it. The juice encourages bile secretion and is valuable in jaundice and gravels — small stones in the urinary tract. The bark of lemon tree is used as a febrifuge to prevent fever and seeds are used as a vermifuge (to expel worms from intestines).

Scurvy

Lemon juice contains more vitamin than the whole fruit, being about 60 mg per 100 gm. The juice also contains appreciable quantity of vitamin B. This makes it an antiscorbutic — an excellent medicine for prevention and treatment of scurvy. A mixture of one part of lemon juice, three parts of water should be taken. Sugar or honey maybe added for taste.

Oral Diseases

With its high vitamin C content lemon helps strengthen both gums and teeth. It is also effective for preventing and curing acute inflammations of the gum margins, pyorrhoea, dental caries and other oral diseases.

Throat Disorders

Lemon is highly beneficial in treatment of throat disorders such as catarrh, choking sensation and itching sensitivities. A ripe unpeeled lemon should be roasted slowly until it begins to crack open. Then one teaspoonful of its juice with a little honey should be taken once every hour, or the juice mixed in a glass of boiled water and flavoured with honey sipped slowly.

Burning Soles and Heels

Lot of toxin elimination takes place through pores of the feet. Rubbing the soles of feet with sliced lemon promotes elimination and keeps the feet free from pain, distress and burning sensation.

Digestive Problems

A ripe lemon is a good appetiser; lemon juice stimulates the flow of saliva and gastric juices and is regarded as an excellent digestive agent. It destroys intestinal worms and eliminates gases formed in the digestive tract. It is highly beneficial for treating digestive problems like dyspepsia, constipation and biliousness. Heartburn is easily relieved by taking juice of half a lemon in a glass of water.

Fevers

Lemon juice makes an effective thirst-quenching drink in pox, measles, scarlet and other fevers which are attendant with extreme thirst and a hot, dry skin. About 15 to 25 gm of lemon juice should be taken in these conditions.

Hemorrhage

Lemon is effective in hemorrhage or bleeding of lungs, stomach, intestines, uterus, kidneys and other internal organs. In such cases, lemon juice with water is advised several times a day.[1]

Spleen Enlargement

Lemon is valuable in the cases of enlarged spleen. Two lemons, cut into halves and heated slightly after adding a little salt, have proved beneficial in this condition.

Rheumatism/Rheumatic Affections

Though lemon juice is sour in taste, its reaction in the body is alkaline and therefore valuable in the treatment of rheumatic affections such as gout, rheumatism, sciatica, lumbago, pain in hip joints which result from too much acid in the body. A sufficient

---

1. K.R. Mukherjee, *Protective Foods in Health and Disease*, pp. 97, Prakritick Chikitsalaya, Calcutta, Fourth Edition, 1983.

intake of lemon juice prevents deposit of uric acid in the tissues and thus reduces the possibility of gout attack.

Obesity

Exclusive intake of lemon juice is an effective remedy for obesity. On the first day the patient should be given nothing but plenty of water. On the second day juice of three lemons mixed with equal amount of water is to be given. One lemon should be subsequently increased each day until till juice of 12 lemons a day is reached. The lemons should then be decreased, one a day, until only three lemons are taken in a day. The patient may feel weak and hungry on the first two days, but the condition stabilises in a few days.

> Healthy eating is your
> one-in-all doctor!
> You can effectively battle & prevent
> disease by consuming healthy food.

Cold

London's first influenza epidemic in November 1931 was cured not by doctors but by lemon. Someone has appropriately said, 'A lemon a day keeps a cold away.' For a bad cold, juice of two lemons in half-a-litre of boiling water, sweetened with honey, taken at bed time, is a very effective remedy.[1]

Circulatory Disorders

Lemon is a rich source of vitamin P; it contains 1.75 mg of this vitamin per 100 gm. It is found both in the juice and peel of the fruit. This vitamin is essential for controlling hemorrhage in a variety of conditions and for preventing capillary fragility. It is, therefore, regarded as a valuable food medicine in high blood pressure and arteriosclerosis. It strengthens the entire arterial system and consequently, is of value in many blood circulatory disorders and heart weakness.

---

1. Dr. S.J. Singh, *Food Remedies*, pp. 116, Nature Cure Council of Medical Research, Lucknow, 1982.

Lemon peel is equally effective in these disorders. Shredded lemon peel may be added to soups and stews, or sprinkled over salad. To make a medicine, peel of one or two lemons are cut finely and kept in warm water for about 12 hours. A teaspoonful may be taken every three hours, or immediately before or after a meal.

Cholera

Lemon has wonderful anti-cholera properties. Lemon juice can kill cholera bacilli within a short time. It is also a very effective and reliable preventive food against cholera during the epidemic. For this purpose, it can be taken in the form of sweetened or salted beverages. Lemon with meals daily also helps keeps cholera away.

Foot Relaxation

Those who walk long distances often get comfort by soaking feet in hot water and then rubbing the feet with lemon juice. The benefit is in the contrasting actions of the hot water which opens the pores and the lemon juice which presents a cooling, astringent action. This treatment with its relaxing action on the foot nerves[1] is also said to promote healthy sleep.

Corn

Lemon is valuable in corns. A fresh slice of lemon tied over the painful area at night and provides relief by morning.

Beauty Aid

Lemon is regarded as a youth restorative. To help cleanse blemished skin, the area should be rubbed with a fresh piece of lemon, and allowed to remain overnight so that it is fully soaked by the skin. Strained fresh lemon juice mixed with cool water and used for washing hair adds to brightness. Dry or scaly skin rubbed with the peel of a lemon restores the skin to softness. Rough elbows can be softened by rubbing with the cut side of a lemon.[2]

---

1. Eric F.W. Powell, *Health from the Kitchen*, pp. 16, Health Science Press, England, 1973.
2. Carlson Wade, *Health Secrets from the Orient*, pp. 133, Allied Publishers Pvt. Ltd., Bombay.

LIME

Botanical Name: *Citrus aurantifolia*
Indian Name: *Niboo*

Lime is an important citrus group fruit. It is considered a health food of great value. It is not to be confused with lemon. Lime and lemon represent two seperate varieties of the same genus. Lime is smaller than lemon and has a thin smooth skin. It has a sweet smell and less juice than a lemon. Lime grows on a small, multi-branched tree with spiny branches, small green leaves and white strongly scented flowers.

It is almost universally used with everyday meals in tropical regions. There are many varieties of lime, differing in size, colour and shape. Limes are classified into two main groups, namely, the sweet and the acid. Sweet limes contain higher proportion of sugar but an insipid taste and are not considered to be of high nutritive value. They are, therefore, not grown on large scale. Acid or sour limes, on the other hand, are extensively cultivated; their importance as food and medicine has been recognised for centuries. The two most popularly known varieties are *Pati* and *Kagzi niboo*.

Origin and Distribution: Lime is believed to have originated in India, where it has been grown since the Vedic times. Arab traders probably took it to Mediterranean and Western countries around 1000 AD. The Spaniards took it to the Americas during colonization. It has since spread throughout the tropics, and is one of the most commonly cultivated species of acid citrus.

Food Value: Acid limes are excellent source of free citric acid, natural sugar, vitamin C, calcium and phosphorus. It contains far more vitamin C than lemon. It is generally taken for its juice in many ways. One of the best ways is to take it with water. Lime juice forms an indispensable ingredient of salads. In fruit salads, it helps to retain the normal colour of fruits and imparts a tart-like flavour. It is often squeezed over cooked pulses, soups, sauces and gravies to make them tastier and palatable.

Lime*

Food Value		Minerals and Vitamins	
Moisture	84.6%	Calcium	90 mg
Protein	1.5%	Phosphorus	20 mg
Fat	1.0%	Iron	0.3 mg
Minerals	0.7%	Vitamin C	63 mg
Fibre	1.3%	Small amounts of	
Carbohydrates	10.9%	Vitamin B Complex	
	100%		

**Values per 100 gms edible portion | Calorific Value - 59*

Natural Benefits and Curative Properties

Juice of fresh limes has been used in traditional Indian medicine since the Vedic times. In the *Vedas*, it has been mentioned as a sacred fruit. Cutting limes after reciting certain *mantras* was believed to drive away evil spirits. *Charaka* and *Sharangdhara*, the famous physicians of ancient India, have mentioned the therapeutic value of lime in various diseases of bones and joints. The vitamin C content in lime increases body's immunity and resistance to fight disease, aids in healing wounds and prevents damage to the eyes. Vitamin C is also helpful in maintaining healthy teeth and strengthening the bones. It prevents tooth decay, dental caries, toothache, bleeding gums and fragility of bones.

The rind of the fruit contains a volatile oil which is used in medicine for improving digestion and eliminating gastric discomfort.

Scurvy

As a rich source of vitamin C, lime has been regarded as a food of exceptional therapeutic value. It has saved the lives of innumerable crews of the ocean-going vessels from scurvy. The Boards of Trade regulations have made it compulsory for the crew to have a supply of lime juice when vegetables are not available.

Digestive Disorders

Lime is highly beneficial in treating digestive disorders. A teaspoonful of fresh lime-juice mixed with equal quantity of honey should be licked to stop bilious vomiting, indigestion, heartburn caused by acidity and for excessive accumulation of saliva in the mouth.

A teaspoonful of lime juice mixed with water and a pinch of soda bicarb makes an excellent remedy for reducing acidity. It also acts as a powerful carminative in case of indigestion. It produces a marked sedative effect in the stomach by releasing carbonic acid gas.[1]

Constipation

Lime juice is of great value in constipation when taken in a glass of warm water first thing in the morning. In chronic cases, it helps remove the disorder by promoting biliary secretion from liver.

Peptic Ulcers

The citric acid in lime has an alkaline reaction in the body. This together with the mineral salts in the juice, help digestion by assisting in the absorption of fats and alcohol, and by neutralising excessive bile produced by the liver. The juice counteracts the effects of greasy food and reduces gastric acidity. It is, therefore, specially valuable in the treatment of peptic ulcers.[2]

Common Cold

Lime is ideal in all types of fevers and colds. Vitamin C in the lime juice increases resistance, reduces toxicity and cuts down the course of illness. Unless allergic, one should not avoid lime in colds. A glass of diluted lime juice in warm water with a teaspoonful of honey added, is an ideal remedy for cold and dry cough.

Tonsillitis

Lime is effective in treating for acute tonsillitis. A fresh lime squeezed in a glass of warm water, with three four teaspoonful of honey and a quarter teaspoonful of common salt, should be sipped slowly in such cases.

Gums

A glass of diluted fresh lime juice mixed with a pinch of rock salt is recommended for healing swollen gums. Squeezed lime rind may also be rubbed on gums before throwing it away.

---

1. Dr. Aman, *Medicinal Secrets of Your Food*, pp. 227-228, IndoAmerican Hospital, Mysore, 1985.
2. Henlen Jeans, *About Tropical Fruits*, pp. 40, Thorsons Publishers Lid., London, 1972.

Gout

The fruit has been used as a remedy in gout and arthritis since long. Vitamin C is known to prevent sore joints by strengthening connective tissues of the body. Citric acid in the lime is a solvent of uric acid which is the primary cause of gout and other diseases of this nature.

Eye Disorders

Few drops of warm lime-juice diluted with water should be instilled in the eyes in case of conjunctivitis. Its regular use with pure rose water in the ratio of 1:4 is helpful in preventing old-age cataract.[1]

Piles, Bleeding

For healing bleeding piles a small lime slit into two, sprinkled with rock salt should be tucked inside the mouth to let the juice flow in. Lime juice with its anti-haemorrhagic properties and rock salt rich in magnesium sulphate, checks bleeding, helps good bowel movement and gradually shrinks the pile mass.

Cystitis

Lime is valuable in cystitis i.e. inflammation of urinary bladder. A teaspoonful of lime juice is mixed with 180 gm of cooled boiled water should be given every two hours in quantities of 60 gm. It gives relief to burning sensation and also stops bleeding in cystitis.

Scorpion Sting

When externally applied, fresh lime is highly beneficial in treatment of scorpion sting. A crystal of potassium permanganate should also be put over it. It will have effect in ten minutes.

Obesity

Fresh juice of one lime stirred in a glassful of water and sweetened with honey taken every morning on empty stomach helps reduce weight within three to four two months. One should also stick to low calorie diet to get the desired result. Lime mixed with honey in warm water also helps to soothe nerves.

---

1. Dr. Aman, *Medicinal Secrets of Your Food*, pp. 229, Indo-American Hospital, Mysore, 1985.

Beauty Aid

Lime can be used as a beauty aid. A fresh lime is squeezed in a glassful of boiled whole milk and a teaspoonful of glycerine added to it. It is left for half an hour and then applied on the face, hands and feet at night. This application at bedtime helps one to look younger and beautiful. This application can also cure pimples, cracked soles and palms, dryness of the face and is a protection against hot and cold winds and sun-burn.

Massaging few drops of lime juice with *amla* juice every night before going to bed, stops hair loss, lengthens hair and prevents premature greying. It also cures dandruff.

Precautions: The alkaline salts of the lime juice neutralises the free uric acid and precipitates it. Excessive may therefore cause formation of renal calculi.

Excessive sucking of fresh lime is also bad for teeth as the acid damages the delicate enamel of the teeth and makes them sensitive. Its excessive use weakens digestion and impoverishes the blood.

MANGO

Botanical Name: *Mangifera indica*
Indian Name: *Aam*

Mango is fruit of the tropics and is called 'king of Asiatic fruits'. It is a fleshy fruit with a thin skin and a central stone containing the seed. It is variable in size and shape, with varying mixtures of green, yellow and red colour. Inside the fruit is stony endocarp of variable size. Mango grows on a large, erect, branched, evergreen tree with deep glossy green leaves. The fruit is used in ceremonial decorations and its dry twigs are used to light sacred fires. The poorer quality of mangoes tend to be fibrous with a turpentine flavour, but the best are juicy, sweet, with very little fibre and a deliciously piquant flavour.

Origin and Distribution: The fruit is indigenous to India. It has been cultivated for over 4000 years. In *Vedas*, mango is praised as a heavenly fruit. In Hindu mythology, it is believed that when Lord Shiva and Parvati came from the Himalayas, they missed this heavenly fruit. Parvati, who was very fond of mango, requested her husband to create a mango tree which Lord Shiva with his divine power fulfilled and mango appeared in India.

Alexander and his men were the first Europeans to see mango in India in 327 BC. It was probably taken to the Malaya region and the East Asian countries by Indians in the fifth century BC and to the East African coast by Persians about 10th century AD.

Mango has numerous varieties; in India alone, there are over 500 varieties, but only about 35 varieties are extensively cultivated.

Food Value: Mango is used as food in all stages of its development. Green or unripe mango contains a large portion of starch which gradually changes into glucose, sucrose and maltose as the fruit begins to ripens and by the time fruit is fully ripe there is no starch left. Green mango is a rich source of pectin which gradually diminishes after formation of the stone. Due to the presence of oxalic, citric, malic and succinic acids unripe mango is sour in taste.

It is a valuable item of diet and a household remedy. Raw mango is a valuable source of vitamin C. It contains more vitamin C than half-ripe or fully ripe mangoes. It is also a good source of vitamin B_1 and B_2 and contains sufficient quantity of niacin. These vitamins differ in concentration in various varieties and during different stages of maturity. Environmental conditions may also affect the vitamin concentration.

Mango*

Food Value		**Minerals and Vitamins**	
Moisture	81.0%	Calcium	14 mg
Protein	0.6%	Phosphorus	16 mg
Fat	0.4%	Iron	1.3 mg
Minerals	0.4%	Vitamin C	16.0%
Fibre	0.7%	Small amounts of	
Carbohydrates	16.9%	Vitamin B Complex	
	100%		

**Values per 100 gms edible portion | Calorific Value - 74*

The ripe fruit is wholesome and nourishing. The chief food ingredient of mango is sugar. The acids contained in the fruit are tartaric and malic acids, besides a trace of citric acid. These acids help to maintain the alkali reserve of the body.

Natural Benefits and Curative Properties

Both ripe and unripe mangoes are known for their medicinal properties. The unripe fruit is acidic, astringent and antiscorbutic, and its skin is an astringent and a stimulant tonic. The bark also has astringent properties with a marked action on mucous membranes.[1] The ripe mango is antiscorbutic, diuretic, laxative, invigorating, fattening and astringent. It tones up the heart muscle, improves complexion and stimulates appetite. It increases the seven body nutrients called *'dhatus'* in Ayurveda. They are food, juice, blood, flesh, fat, bone marrow and semen. The fruit is beneficial in liver disorders, loss of weight and other physical disturbances.

Mango pickles are used throughout India. However, these pickles, if extremely sour, spicy and oily, are not good for health and should be avoided by those suffering from arthritis, rheumatism, sinusitis, sore throat and hyperacidity.

Unripe Mango

Heat Stroke

Unripe mangoes protect against the effects of hot, scorching summer winds. A drink prepared from an unripe mangoes by cooking in hot ashes and mixing the pith with sugar and water, is an effective remedy for heat exhaustion and heat stroke. Eating raw mangoes with salt quenches thirst and prevents excessive loss of sodium chloride and iron resulting from excessive sweating.

Gastroentritis

Unripe green mangoes are beneficial in treating gastro-intestinal disorders. Eating one or two small tender mangoes with salt and honey is an effective medicine for summer diarrhoea, dysentery,

---

1. J.F. Dartur, *Medicinal Plants of India & Pakistan*, pp. 106, D.B. Taraporevala Sons & Co. (P) Ltd., Bombay, 1985.

piles, morning sickness, chronic dyspepsia, indigestion and constipation.[1]

Bilious Disorders

Unripe mangoes are an excellent remedy for bilious disorders. The acids contained in the green mango increase secretion of bile and act as intestinal antiseptic. Eating a green mango daily with honey and pepper cures biliousness, food putrefaction, urticaria and hepatitis or jaundice. It tones up the liver and keeps it healthy.[2]

Blood Disorders

The high concentration of vitamin C in green mangoes increases the elasticity of blood vessels and helps in formation of new blood cells. It aids in absorption of food-iron and prevents bleeding tendencies. It increases resistance against tuberculosis, anaemia, cholera and dysentery.

Scurvy

Amchur, a popular kitchen item in Indian houses, consists of green mangoes skinned, stoned, cut into pieces and sun dried. On account of its citric content, 15 gm of *amchur* is said to be equivalent to 30 gm of good lime. It is valuable in treating scurvy.[3]

Ripe Mango

Eye Disorders

Ripe mangoes are highly beneficial in the treatment of night blindness — the inability to see properly in dim light which results from deficiency of vitamin A. Liberal use of mangoes also prevents many other eye diseases which may ultimately cause total blindness, prevent development of refractive errors, dryness of eyes, softening of the cornea, itching and burning in the eyes.[4]

---

1. Hakeem Rasool Sahib, *Jiryan-Ka-illaj*, (Urdu Mss.) 289, Mandi Mohalla, Mysore, 1930.
2. Hakeem Mahboob Ali Khan Bakshi, *Amm-say-Bimarioon-ka Illaj*, (Urdu Mss.) Mandi Mohalla, Mysore, 1959.
3. Dr. S.J. Singh, *Food Remedies*, pp. 128, Nature Cure Council of Medical Research, Lucknow, 1982.
4. Dr. Aman, *Medicinal Secrets of Your Food*, pp. 256, Indo-American Hospital, Mysore, 1985.

Infections

All bacterial invasions are due to poor epithelium, the tissue that covers the external surface of the body. Liberal use of mangoes in season helps formation of healthy epithelium, thereby preventing frequent attacks of common infections such as colds, rhinitis and sinusitis due to high concentration of vitamin A.

Loss of Weight

A combination of mangoes and milk is ideal for weight loss. Ripe and sweet mangoes should be taken thrice a day — morning, noon and evening followed by milk. Mangoes are rich in sugar but deficient in protein. On the other hand, milk is rich in protein but deficient in sugar. Thus one complements the other.

Diabetes

An infusion prepared from tender leaves of mango tree is effective in controlling diabetes. This infusion is prepared from fresh leaves by soaking them overnight in water and squeezing them in water the next morning before filtering the water. As an alternative to infusion, leaves can be dried in shade, powdered and preserved. Half a teaspoonful of this powder twice a day, morning and evening, is advised.

Diarrhoea

Mango seeds collected during the mango growing season are valuable in diarrhoea. The seeds are dried in shade, powdered and stored for use as medicine. This powder should be given in doses of about one and a half gram to two grams with or without honey. Juice of fresh flowers when taken with one or two teaspoonful of curd, is also valuable in treating diarrhoea.

Female Disorders

Mango seeds are considered useful in some disorders of female reproductive organs. According to Dr. Aman, 'A teaspoonful of paste of the decorticated kernel of mango is applied inside the vagina to cure leucorrhoea, vaginitis and relaxed walls caused by multiple pregnancies. Its application half an hour before intercourse gives a virgin feeling and acts as a safe contraceptive. This has been often been tried with gratifying results.'[1]

Juice of the fresh mango bark is valuable in heavy bleeding during menstruation, i.e. menorrhagia, leucorrhoea, mucus and pus discharges from the uterus and bleeding or hemorrhage from uterus. The juice is given after adding egg white or some mucilage — a kind of vegetable glue obtained from plant — and a little opium. In the alternative, a mixture of 10 ml of a fluid extract of the bark and 120 ml of water is given in doses of a teaspoonful every hour or two.

Throat Disorders

Mango bark is effective in treating diphtheria and throat diseases. Its fluid is locally applied and also used as a gargle. The gargle is prepared by mixing 10 ml of fluid extract with 125 ml of water.

Scorpion Bites/Bee Sting

Applying the juice which oozes out at the time of plucking the fruit gives immediate relief to pain from scorpion bite or the sting of a bee. The juice can be collected and kept in a bottle.

Precautions: Excessive intake of unripened mangoes may cause throat irritation, indigestion, dysentery and abdominal colic. Not more than one or two green mangoes should be taken daily. Water should not to be taken immediately after eating a green mango because it coagulates the sap and makes it an irritant. Sap or milky juice which comes out on breaking the stalk of the green mango is an irritant and an astringent. Eating green mangoes without draining the sap may cause mouth, throat and gastro intestinal irritation. The sap should, therefore be fully squeezed out or the skin should be peeled before using raw mango.

Excessive eating of mangoes may produce ailments like constipation, eye affections, blood impurities and seasonal fever and children can suffer from skin disease in season.

---

1. Dr. Aman, *Clinical Observation of Mango Kernal on the Mortality of Sperms and its Spermicidal Action*, pp. 120, 1962-67.

ORANGE

Botanical Name: *Citrus aurantium*
Indian Name: *Santrā*

Orange is one of the finest gifts of nature. It is perhaps the most popular and wide-spread of citrus fruits. It is a delicious and a nourishing fruit which is upto 12 cm in diameter, though most common varieties are smaller in diameter. The fruit grows on a spreading evergreen tree with dark green leaves and fragrant flowers.

The more important varieties of oranges are the loose-skinned oranges, the tight-skinned oranges and the sour-oranges; loose-skinned variety is popular in India and the tight-skinned in Europe.

Origin and Distribution: Orange is a native of the south China region. It is believed to have travelled to India from where it was taken to the west by Vasco da Gama in 1498. In India, the loose-skinned orange variety grows widely in some regions of Maharashtra, the Coorg region in Karnataka and in Assam.

Food Value: Orange is a rich source of protective food ingredients like vitamins A, B, C and calcium. As a source of calcium it is superior to almost any other fruit. Orange also contains sodium, potassium, magnesium, copper, sulphur and chlorine.

Its vitamin C content helps the body tissues to use the calcium.

Orange*

Food Value		**Minerals and Vitamins**	
Moisture	87.6%	Calcium	26 mg
Protein	0.7%	Phosphorus	20 mg
Fat	0.2%	Iron	0.3 mg
Minerals	0.3%	Vitamin C	30 mg
Fibre	0.3%	Small amounts of	
Carbohydrates	10.9%	Vitamin B Complex	
	100%		

**Values per 100 gms edible portion | Calorific Value - 59*

Natural Benefits and Curative Properties

Orange is a pre-digested food; the starch content of oranges is converted into readily assimilable sugar in sunshine and soon absorbed in the blood.

Regular use of orange prevents frequent attacks of common cold, influenza and bleeding tendencies. It keeps one healthy and contributes towards longevity. Orange juice can be given in most dieases.

Fevers

Orange is an excellent food in all types of fever when the digestive power is seriously impaired. The patient may suffer from blood poisoning called toxaemia and the lack of saliva coats the tongue and often destroys thirst for water and desire for food. The agreeable flavour of orange juice helps greatly in overcoming these drawbacks. Orange juice is an ideal food in fevers like typhoid, tuberculosis and measles. It gives energy, increases urinary output and promotes resistance against infections thereby hastening recovery.

Dyspepsia

Orange is an effective remedy in chronic dyspepsia. It gives rest to the digestive organs and supplies nutrition in its most easily assimilable form. It also stimulates the flow of digestive juices thereby stimulating appetite. It creates a suitable condition for the growth of friendly bacteria in the intestines.

Constipation

The general stimulating influence of orange juice excites peristaltic activity and helps prevent accumulation of food residue in the colon, which leads to putrefaction and auto-intoxication.[1]

Diseases of Bone and Teeth

As an excellent source of calcium and vitamin C, orange is valuable in diseases of bone and teeth. Disorders in the structure of the teeth usually result from shortage of vitamin C and calcium; these can be overcome by sufficient intake of orange. Dr. Harke, a Chicago

---

1. Dr. S.J. Singh, *Food Remedies*, pp. 152, Nature Cure Council of Medical Research, Lucknow, 1982.

physician, has claimed to have cured several patients of pyorrhoea and dental caries with large amounts of orange juice.[1]

Children's Ailments

Orange juice is considered an excellent food for infants not fed on breast milk. They should be given 15 ml to 120 ml of orange juice daily according to age. It prevents scurvy and rickets and helps growth. This juice can also be given with beneficial results to more grown up babies whose normal development may be unsatisfactory.[2]

Heart Disease

Orange juice, sweetened with honey, is highly beneficial in heart diseases. In cardiac conditions like coronary ischemia and infarction, when only liquid food is advisable, orange juice with honey is a safe energy giving liquid food.[3]

Orange Peels are full of powerful antioxidants

According to a study in the *Journal of Agriculture and Food Chemistry,* 2004, powerful antioxidants called super flavonoids found in orange and tangerine peels can reduce levels of bad LDL cholesterol, without lowering the good cholesterol HDL levels. Antioxidants from the peel were 20 times more powerful than those from the juice. 'The same goes for all citrus fruits,' says award winning nutritionist and international author Anita Bean. 'Although we throw away the peel because of their bitter taste, the pith contains high levels of pectin, a component of dietary fibre known to help lower cholesterol.'

How to eat it: Add grated orange peel to salads, cauliflower or any baked vegetable to add tang.

1. J.B.S. Braverman, *Citrus Products,* pp. 3, Interscience Publishers, Inc, New York, 1949.
2. K.R. Mukherjee, *Protective Foods in Health & Disease,* pp. 136, Prakritick Chikitsalaya, Calcutta, 1983.
3. Dr. Aman, *Medicinal Secrets of Your Food,* pp. 237, Indo-American Hospital, Mysore, 1985.

Difficult Expectorations

Orange juice mixed with a pinch of salt and a tablespoonful of honey is an effective remedy for tuberculosis, asthma, common cold, bronchitis and cough associated with difficult expectorations. Due to its saline action in the lungs, it eases expectorations and protects from secondary infection.

Acne

Orange peel, pounded well with water on a piece of stone, should be applied to the affected areas to treat acne.

Uses

Orange is used in a variety of ways. It is usually taken as a dessert fruit. Large quantities of the fruit are used for canned orange juice. It is also made into squashes and used for marmalades and jams. Essential oil from the rind of the fruit is valued in perfumery.

PAPAYA

Botanical Name: *Carica papaya*
Indian Name: *Papitā*

Papaya is one of the most valuable of all tropical fruits. It is a large, fleshy, hollow berry upto 50-60 cm in diameter and usually weighs from ½ kg to 2 kg. It is cylindrical or pear-shaped. The central cavity is surrounded by hundreds of small seeds, though sometimes seedless varieties are available.

The fruit has a thin smooth skin. As the papaya ripens the skin colour changes from green to bright yellowish or orange colour. Inside, the thick juicy yellow or pink flesh, has a soft melting quality. It has a delicate aroma and is delicious to eat.

Origin and Distribution: Papaya appears to have originated in southern Mexico and Costa Rica. It was taken by the Spaniards to the Philippines in the mid-16th century and gradually spread to all tropical and sub-tropical countries. It is now widely cultivated in Indian sub-continent, China, Mexico, Brazil, Peru, Venezuela, Central and South Africa, Philippines, Australia and Pacific islands.

Food Value: Papaya is as a wholesome fruit. The daily requirements of some essential nutrients like proteins, mineral and vitamins can be met from this fruit. The vitamin C contents in papaya increases as it ripens. Its carbohydrate content is mostly invert sugar which is a form of pre-digested food.

Papaya*

Food Value		**Minerals and Vitamins**	
Moisture	90.8%	Calcium	17 mg
Protein	0.6%	Phosphorus	13 mg
Fat	0.1%	Iron	0.5 mg
Minerals	0.5%	Vitamin C	57 mg
Fibre	0.8%	Small amounts of	
Carbohydrates	7.2%	Vitamin B Complex	
	100%		

**Values per 100 gms edible portion | Calorific Value - 32*

Natural Benefits and Curative Properties

Papaya has remarkable medicinal virtues which were fully recognised even in the ancient times. It is not only one of the most easily digested fruits, but also aids in digestion of other foods. Ripe papaya is an excellent tonic for growing children, for pregnant women and nursing mothers. It is an energy giving food.

Digestive Aid

Modern scientific investigations into the properties of papaya have confirmed many of the ancient beliefs about its virtues. The most important of these is the discovery of a protein digesting enzyme in the milky juice or latex. The enzyme is similar to pepsin in digestive action and is reputed to be so powerful that it can digest 200 times its own weight in protein. Its effect is to assist the body's own enzymes in assimilating the maximum nutritional value from food for providing energy and bodybuilding materials.[1]

1. Henlen Jeans, *About Tropical Fruits*, pp. 49, Thorsons Publishers Ltd, London, 1972.

Intestinal Disorders

Papain in raw papaya is highly beneficial in making up the deficiency of gastric juice, excess of unhealthy mucus in the stomach, in dyspepsia and in intestinal irritation. The ripe fruit, if eaten regularly, corrects habitual constipation, bleeding piles and chronic diarrhoea. The juice of the papaya seeds is also useful in dyspepsia and bleeding piles.[1]

Roundworms

The digestive enzyme papain in the milky juice of unripe papaya is a powerful anthelmintic (i.e. which has the power to destroy) for roundworms. A tablespoonful of fresh juice mixed with an equal quantity of honey taken with three to four tablespoonful of hot water is the suggested dose for an adult. This dose should be followed two hours later with 30 to 60 ml of castor oil mixed in 250-375 ml of luke warm milk. For children of 7 to 10 years, only half the above doses should be given. For children under three years, a teaspoonful is sufficient.

Papaya seeds are rich in a substance called caricin which is an effective medicine for expelling roundworms. The alkaloid carpaine found in the leaves has also the power to destroy or expel intestinal worms. They are given with honey.

Skin Disorders

Juice of the raw papaya is an irritant and useful in several skin disorders. It can be applied with benefit to skin swellings for preventing formation of pus or suppuration and to corns, warts, pimples, horn, an excrescence or an abnormal growth of skin and other skin diseases. As a cosmetic, it removes freckles or brown spots caused by exposure to sunlight leaving the skin smooth and delicate. A paste of papaya seeds is applied in skin diseases like ringworm.

Menstrual Irregularities

Unripe papaya helps the contraction of the muscle fibres of the womb and is therefore beneficial in securing proper menstrual flow.

---

1. J.F. Dastur, *Medicinal Plants of India and Pakistan*, pp. 47, D.B. Taraporevala & Sons & Co. (P) Ltd., Bombay, 1985.

It is especially helpful in case of cessation of menstruation resulting from exposure to cold or due to fright in young girls.

Cirrhosis of the liver

Black seeds of papaya are highly beneficial in treatment of cirrhosis of the liver caused by alcoholism, malnutrition etc. A tablespoonful of juice obtained by grinding the seeds, mixed with ten drops of fresh lime juice, should be given once or twice daily for about a month as a medicine for this disease.[1]

Throat Disorders

Fresh juice of raw papaya mixed with honey can be applied with beneficial results over inflamed tonsils (tonsillitis) for diphtheria and other throat disorders. It dissolves the membrane and prevents infection from spreading.

Spleen Enlargement

Ripe papaya is highly valuable in cases of enlarged spleen. The fruit should be skinned, cut into pieces and immersed in vinegar for a week. About 20 gms of the fruit thus preserved should be consumed twice with meals in the treatment of this disease.[2] Slices of peeled raw fruit with cumin seeds and pepper can also be used once daily to cure enlarged spleen due to malaria.

Uses

Papaya is used in a variety of ways. The ripe fresh fruits are taken with breakfast, dessert, and in fruit salads. They are used for making soft drinks, jams and in flavouring ice creams. Unripe fruits are generally taken as a vegetable.

Papain, prepared from the dried latex of immature fruits is used to make the meat tender, to manufacture chewing-gum, in cosmetics and as a drug for digestive ailments.

---

1. Dr. Aman, *Medicinal Secrets of Your Food*, pp. 273, Indo-American Hospital, Mysore, 1985.
2. Hakeem H. Abdul Hameed Saheb, *The Complete Book of Home Remedies*, pp. 116, Orient Paperbacks, Delhi, 1988.

POMEGRANATE

Botanical Name: *Punica granatum*
Indian Name: *Anār*

Pomegranate is a delicious semi-seedy fruit. It has refreshing and soothing qualities and is easier to digest than most other fruit. The fruit has been held in high esteem both as a food and a medicine since time immemorial. It is a symbol of plenty. Pomegranate is a six-sided fruit of fairly large size with tough leathery skin. It is divided inside into several cells containing numerous angular seeds. These seeds are surrounded by a succulent coating of pink or crimson colour with a delicious sub-acid flavour. The sweet ruby-pink and the sour varieties are most popular.

Origin and Distribution: Pomegranate is a native of Iran and Afghanistan. It was grown in the hanging gardens of Babylon and was known to ancient Egyptians. It spread early around the Mediterranean and eastwards to India, China and Japan. In India, it is cultivated mostly in Maharashtra, Gujarat and to a limited extent in Uttar Pradesh.

Pomegrante*

Food Value		**Minerals and Vitamins**	
Moisture	78.0%	Calcium	10 mg
Protein	1.6%	Phosphorus	70 mg
Fat	0.1%	Iron	0.3 mg
Minerals	0.7%	Vitamin C	16 mg
Fibre	5.1%	Small amounts of	
Carbohydrates	14.5%	Vitamin B Complex	
	100%		

**Values per 100 gms edible portion | Calorific Value - 65*

Curative and Medicinal Properties

Pomegranate has been regarded as a food medicine of great value. All parts of the tree, the roots, the reddish brown bark, leaves, flowers, rind and seeds, have featured in medicine for thousands of years. Medical practitioners of ancient India have described it as a light food and a tonic for the heart. The medical writers of ancient

Arabia regarded it as a fruit good for inflammation of the stomach and for heart pain. Sweet varieties of the fruit are considered a good laxative, while those intermediate between sweet and sour are regarded as valuable in stomach inflammations and heart pain.[1]

Juice of fresh fruit is an excellent cooling beverage for alleviating thirst in fevers and sickness. It acts on the liver, heart and kidneys and tones up their functions. It supplies the required minerals and helps the liver to preserve vitamin A from the food. It increases resistance against infections, particularly tuberculosis.

Digestive Disorders

Pomegranate juice is of great value in digestive disorders. It is an appetiser, aids digestion and is useful for patients suffering from colitis and mucous. It binds the stool and tones up the intestines. A tablespoonful of the juice mixed with equal quantity of honey can be given with beneficial results in bilious vomiting i.e. bile containing fluid and nausea, burning in the chest due to excessive secretion of bile, flatulent colic and morning sickness.

Diarrhoea and Dysentery

The astringent property of pomegranate is of great value — it causes cells to shrink and is a valuable food medicine for diarrhoea and dysentery. Pomegranate juice about 50 ml is given repeatedly to patients who develop weakness on account of profuse and continuous purging. This helps control diarrhoea. Fresh pomegranate juice also stops passing of blood with stool. The flower buds of the plant are astringent and useful in the treatment of chronic diarrhoea and dysentery, especially of children.[2]

Intestinal Worms

The bark, the root and the stem of pomegranate tree, are well known for its anthelmintic properties of destroying parasitic worms. However, root-bark is preferred as it contains greater quantity of the alkaloid punicine than the stem-bark. This alkaloid is highly

---

1. Helen Jeans, *About Tropical Fruits*, pp. 68, Thorsons Publishers Ltd. London, 1972.
2. J.F. Dastur, *Medicinal Plants of India and Pakistan*, pp. 139, D.B. Taraporevala Sons & Co. (P) Ltd., Bombay, 1985.

toxic to tape worms. A cold decoction prepared preferably of fresh bark, is suggested thrice a day in doses of 90 to 180 ml at intervals of one hour to an adult. A purgative should be given after the last dose. The dose for children is 30 to 60 ml. The decoction is also used for expelling tapeworms.[1]

Fevers

Pomegrante juice, with a little saffron added, is useful in fevers to allay thirst. A *sherbet* of the ripe fruit is beneficial in treatment of typhus, gastric and asthmatic fevers. The root bark is also given as a febrifuge to prevent fevers.[2]

Anal Itching

The skin of the pomegranate fruit is considered highly beneficial in treatment of anal itching. This nasty discomfort may result from unhygienic habits or worm infection. The skin of the fruit should be roasted till it is brittle and black, then powdered and mixed with a little vegetable oil, and applied over the anus for relief.

Kidney and Bladder Stones

Seeds of sour and sweet pomegranate are useful as a medicine. A tablespoonful of seeds, ground into a fine paste given with a cupful of horse-gram soup helps dissolves gravel in kidneys and bladder.

Teeth and Gum Disorder

Powder of the dry rind mixed with pepper and common salt makes for a very good dentifrice i.e. tooth paste or powder. Its regular application strengthens gums, stops bleeding, prevents pyorrhoea, cleans and preserves the teeth.

Uses

Pomegranate is used as a table-fruit. Its juice is regarded as a delicacy and makes an excellent *sherbet*. The fruit is also used in preparing syrups, ice-creams, jellies and jams. Pomegranate has a very good keeping quality and can be kept for about six months in

---

1. Ibid., pp. 139-140.
2. Dr. Aman, *Medicinal Secrets of Your Food*, p. 282, Indo-American Hospital, Mysore, 1985.

cold storage. Its thick rind protects its succulent seeds from much rough handling.

Precautions: The fruit should be eaten soon after it is cut open as the seeds tend to lose colour quickly. Pips should not be swallowed while eating the fruit; it is said to adversly effect the intestines and may cause appendicitis.

RAISINS

Botanical Name: *Vitis vinifera*
Indian Name: *Munaqqa*

Raisins are dried grapes. All grapes however, are, not suitable for converting to raisins, only the very sweet are selected for drying.

Origin and Distribution: Raisins were known to the traders of the Mediterranean even in Greek and Roman ages. Most world production of raisins comes from Italy, France, Spain, Turkey, Iran, Afghanistan, the US Australia and South Africa.

Food Value: Raisins are valued for their food value and nourishing qualities. They are rich in carbohydrates, minerals and vitamins and constitute a valuable food when taken with milk. The two complement each other; milk contains protein and raisins sugar. They also complement nuts like cashewnut, walnut and groundnut.

Raisins*

Food Value		**Minerals and Vitamins**	
Moisture	20.2%	Calcium	87 mg
Protein	1.8%	Phosphorus	80 mg
Fat	0.3%	Iron	7.7 mg
Minerals	2.0%	Vitamin C	1 mg
Fibre	1.1%	Small amounts of	
Carbohydrates	74.6%	Vitamin B Complex	
	100%		

**Values per 100 gms edible portion | Calorific Value - 308*

Raisins are extensively used in salads. They are added to curries, used in bakeries and confectionaries, and widely used in jams, jellies, cakes, puddings and pies.

Natural Benefits and Curative Properties

Raisins contain eight times more sugar than grapes. Like that of the grapes, sugar in the raisins is of superior quality, as major portion is formed by glucose and fruit sugar. Glucose produces quick heat and energy in the body. Raisins are thus an excellent food in all cases of debility and wasting diseases. They are also valuable during convalescence.

In Europe, persons suffering from chronic ailments sometimes recourse to an exclusive diet of raisins for short periods of time. This

> Those who have no time for healthy eating will sooner or later have to find time for illness.
> Edward Stanley

treatment is known as 'raisin cure'. It is believed that raisins taken for one month can bring considerable improvement in health.[1]

Acidosis

Raisins with their high alkalinity, are helpful in maintaining acid balance when acidity is high. Studies done by Saywell at the University of California have shown that the free use of raisins, say about 1.05 gm daily, greatly helps reduce acidity of the urine. Urinary ammonia also gets reduced. The organic acid of the raisins is completely oxidized. The free use of raisins is valuable in combating chronic acidosis which generally results from the excessive consumption of meat and cereals.[2]

---

1. K.R. Mukherjee, *Protective Foods in Health & Disease*, pp. 175, Prakritick Chikitsalaya, Calcutta, 1983.
2. Dr. S.J. Singh, *Food Remedies*, pp. 101, Nature Cure Council of Medical Research, Lucknow, 1982.

Constipation

Raisins are highly beneficial in treating constipation. Soaked in a glassful of drinking water for 24 to 48 hours they should be eaten early morning after discarding the stones. The water in which raisins have been soaked should also be drunk. Taken every morning it brings excellent results in chronic constipation.

As an extract of water in which raisins have been soaked can be given even to infants for regular bowel action. The extract is prepared thus: depending on the child's age, six to ten raisins or more, are soaked in boiling water and cooled. The raisins are then thoroughly crushed to extract their juice in the water. For children, the liquid must be strained for raisin skin before being administered.

Anaemia

As a rich source of easily assimilable iron, raisins enrich blood and are therefore useful in anaemia.

Under Weight

Raisins are a good food for those who wish to gain weight. They may be taken upto 1 kg daily, 30 gm or so at a time.

Febrile Cases

An extract from raisins acts like a medicine in febrile cases i.e. relating to fever. This extract is prepared by soaking raisins in water and crushing them in the same water. The water is then strained and the skin discarded. The raisin water thus prepared becomes a tonic. A little lime juice added to it enhances taste and usefulness.

Sexual Debility

In Ayurveda, black raisins are used for restoring sexual vigour. After washing them thoroughly in lukewarm water they are boiled with milk. This makes them swell and sweet. These raisins are taken with milk. The suggested dosage is to start with 30 gms of raisins with 200 ml of milk, three times daily. The quantity of raisins can then be gradually increased to 50 gms each time.

IMPORTANCE OF VEGETABLES

Vegetables are an important protective food with several important ingredients for building and repairing the body.

Food Value: Vegetables are important for maintaining alkaline reserve in the body. They are rich in vitamin A, B and C and valued for their mineral content. Faulty cooking techniques and careless storage can destroy these valuable elements.

There are different kinds of vegetables — edible roots, stems, leaves, fruits and seeds. Each group contributes to a wholesome and nutritious diet. Fleshy roots are high in energy and a good source of B group vitamins. Seeds are relatively high in carbohydrates and proteins. Leaves, stems and fruits are excellent sources of minerals, vitamins, water and roughage.

It is not that only green vegetables are useful. Farinaceous vegetables consisting of starchy roots such as potatoes, sweet potatoes, the tubers and legumes are equally valuable. They are excellent sources of carbohydrates and provide energy to the body.

Natural Benefits of Vegetables

Most vegetables are best consumed in their raw state as salads. Vegetables used in salads should be fresh, crisp and completely dry. If vegetables have to be cooked, care should be taken to preserve their nutritive value.

An intake of about 280 gms of vegetables per day per person is considered essential for maintaining good health. Of this, leafy vegetables should constitute 40 per cent, roots and tubers 30 per cent, and the other vegetables like brinjal, ladyfingers (okra) the remaining 30 per cent.

Vitamins

Carotene: Many vegetables contain carotene which is converted into vitamin A in the body. Vitamin A is essential for growth and vitality, for good eye-sight, healthy skin and for protection against diseases, especially of the respiratory tract. Deficiency of vitamin A can lead to eye infection, poor vision, night blindness, frequent colds, lack of appetite and skin disorders. Generally, deep green, yellow and orange coloured vegetables such as green leafy vegetables, carrots, papaya tomatoes and yellow pumpkin are rich sources of carotene.

Vitamin B-Complex: Several leafy vegetables like fenugreek leaves, turnip greens and beet green contain riboflavin, a member of the vitamin B-complex. This vitamin is essential for growth, general health of eyes, skin, nails and hair. A deficiency can lead to cracking of the angles of the mouth, premature wrinkles and eczema.

Vitamin C: Vegetables like Indian gooseberry, bitter gourd, tomatoes and leafy vegetables like spinach, cabbage and drumstick leaves are rich in vitamin C. Generally, fresh vegetables are better sources of vitamin C than dried, stale or withered ones. Vitamin C is essential for normal growth and maintenance of body tissues, especially those of the joints, bones, teeth and gums and for protection against infection. A deficiency of this vitamin can lead to scurvy, tooth decay, bleeding gums, anaemia and premature ageing.

Minerals

Vegetables contain highly soluble minerals like calcium, phosphorus, iron, magnesium, copper and potassium all of which help maintain the acid-base balance of the hydrogen concentration of body issues. They assist in complete absorption of vitamins, proteins, fats and carbohydrates from the food. They also help the body to eliminate excess liquid and salt. The diuretic action of vegetables like potato, beans, spinach, radish, turnip and brinjal are specially important in cases of edema or swellings, kidney and heart conditions.

Two important minerals, calcium and iron, are found in vegetables. Calcium is essential for strong bones and teeth. Iron is needed for blood formation. It is an essential constituent of haemoglobin. Calcium and iron are aplenty in leafy vegetables like spinach and fenugreek leaves. Carrot, bitter gourd, onions and tomatoes are also good sources of iron.

Vegetable juices

Fresh raw vegetables juices are rich source of nutritional enzymes and other elements needed by the cells and tissues of the body. While the body can also derive these elements from whole vegetables, but they are more easily digested and assimilated when taken from fresh juices. Vitamin and mineral deficiency can be made up more quickly from fresh juices than by eating raw vegetables.

Practically all vegetables make good juices. These juices may be divided into three main types.

1. Juices from vegetable fruits, that is, tomatoes and cucumber.
2. Juices from green leafy vegetables such as cabbage, celery, lettuce, spinach and parsley, and
3. Juices from root vegetables like beetroot, carrot, onion, potato and radish.

In most cases it is desirable to use juice individually; more than three juices should never be combined. The broad rules applicable in mixing vegetable juices are that juices from vegetable fruits may be combined with those of the green leafy vegetables, but not juices of root vegetables. Juices of green leafy vegetables may be combined with those of root vegetables.

Vegetable juices soothe jaded nerves and gently carry away toxic matter and accumulated waste products. They are best taken at least half an hour or more after meals, never before any meal. Many common ailments respond favourably to raw vegetable juices. Vegetable and fruit juice should never be taken together.

Curative Value

Vegetables contain various therapeutic agents. Vegetables like onion, radish and celery exercise a tonic effect and are excellent for

Tips for Healthy Cooking

1. Wash thoroughly and cut vegetables into large pieces.
2. Add cut vegetables in salt dissolved water and bring to a boiling point. This helps avoid loss of vitamin B-complex and vitamin C.
3. In cooking, use just enough water to cover vegetables. Spinach and other tender greens need no water.
4. Vegetables should be covered tightly while cooking.
5. Cook vegetables for least possible time and only till they are soft to touch. Cooking longer in large quantities of water decreases the nutritive and medicinal value.
6. To prevent loss of nutrients always steam or boil vegetables in their own juices and on a slow fire; water or the cooking liquid should not be drained off.
7. In most root vegetables, the largest amount of minerals is directly under the skin and these are lost if vegetables are peeled.
8. Do not peel vegetables unless so old that peels are hard and unpalatable.
9. To preserve taste and nutrition avoid soaking vegetables.
10. Vegetables should not be cooked in aluminium vessels. Aluminium is a soft metal and is acted upon both by food acids and alkalis. Scientific evidence shows that tiny particles of aluminium from foods cooked in such utensils enters the stomach and the strong astringent properties of aluminium injure the sensitive lining of the stomach which can lead to gastric irritation and digestive and intestinal ailments.
11. Serve cooked vegetables hot.

the nerves. Carrots are good for the blood. White crisp juicy stalks of celery serve is a good medicine in cases of rheumatism or nervous dyspepsia than any other nervine that relieves nerve disorder. A dish of spinach or dandelion is beneficial in treating kidney problems. Lettuce is a good food remedy for insomnia. Onion can be used with advantage in treating cough, cold, influenza, constipation, scurvy and hydrophobia. Leaves of fenugreek are highly valuable in treatment of indigestion, flatulence and sluggish liver. Garlic can be beneficially used in heart diseases, hypertension, hypoglycaemia, diabetes and even in potentially fatal form of meningitis. It has been effectively used in lowering blood cholesterol and preventing blood clotting.

Gastro-Intestinal Disorders

Fibres in vegetables act as mechanical intestinal expanders and help in easy expulsion of body waste. They help to prevent constipation and keep the intestinal tract free from harmful germs. Fibre in the form of cellulose helps in lowering cholesterol level. Beetroot, cabbage, carrots, cucumbers, green peas and beans are equally valuable. They are also useful in cases of arteriosclerosis, high blood pressure and constipation. But if there is inflammation in intestines, vegetables with lower cellulose content such as tomatoes, lettuce, potatoes and vegetable juices should be taken.

Pectin found in vegetables such as brinjal, radish, pumpkin and beetroot absorb water, kill certain bacteria and eliminate toxins from the body. Garlic, onion, radish and mint contain pectin as well as anti-microbic qualities.

Blood Disorders

Vegetables also supply trace elements essential for human organism. Iodine, for instance, is essential for thyroid hormone which regulates much physical and mental activities, cobalt for increasing the number of blood corpuscles, and zinc for proper growth.

AMARANTH

Botanical Name: *Amaranathus gangeticus*
Indian Name: *Chaulai-ka-saag*

Amaranth is a powerhouse of iron, vitamins and minerals. It is a warm season crop grown in summer and rainy season. It the best way of fueling up the seasons best offering. There are about six different species in cultivation.

Resembling spinach in appearance, amaranth leaves come in range from purple to red to green or gold in colur and are found in foothills of the Himalayas to the coast of South India.

Amaranth*

Food Value		**Minerals and Vitamins**	
Moisture	85.7%	Calcium	397 mg
Protein	4.0%	Phosphorus	83 mg
Fat	0.5%	Iron	25.5 mg
Minerals	2.7%	Vitamin C	99 mg
Fibre	1.0%	Small amounts of	
Carbohydrates	6.1%	Vitamin B Complex	
	100%		

**Values per 100 gms edible portion | Calorific Value - 45*

Natural Benefits and Curative Properties

Regular use of amaranth in food prevents deficiency of vitamins A, B_1, B_2, and C, calcium, iron and potassium. It protects against defective vision, respiratory infections, recurrent colds, retarded growth and functional sterility.

Respiratory Disorders

Fresh amaranth juice along with honey is a remedy for chronic bronchitis, asthma, emphysema and tuberculosis.[1]

Pregnancy and Lactation

One cup of fresh leaf juice mixed with honey and a pinch of cardamom powder is recommended during entire term of

1. Dr. Aman, *Medicinal Secrets of Your Foods*, pp. 316, IndoAmerican Hospital, Mysore, 1985.

pregnancy. This helps in normal growth of foetus, prevents loss of calcium and iron, relaxes the uterine ligaments and facilitates easy delivery. Post child birth it shortens the laying-in period, checks complications and increases the flow of breast milk.[1]

Growth in Children

A teaspoonful of fresh juice mixed with few drops of honey given once daily to infants a fortnight after birth helps healthy and strong growth, prevents constipation and eases the teething process.

For growing children this juice is a natural protein tonic. It contains all essential amino-acids such as arginine, histidine, isoleucine, leucine, lysine, cystine, methionine, phenylalanine, threonine, tryptophan and valine.

Premature Ageing

Regular use of amaranth prevents premature ageing. It prevents any disturbance of calcium and iron metabolism which usually occurs in old age. According to Dr. Van-Sylke, calcium molecules begin to get deposited in the bone tissues with age. This haphazard calcium distribution is influenced by improper molecular movements of iron in the tissues. If this molecular disturbance of calcium and iron is prevented by regular supply of calcium and iron as found in amaranth, the process of ageing can be significantly slowed down.

The Powerhouse !

According to Ayurveda, the juice extracted from amaranth leaves is packed with carbohydrates, proteins, minerals and vitamins, and its regular consumption helps in easing digestion, excessive menstruation and weight management. Since it is high in iron content and dietary fibre, it is good for anaemic patients, and reduces cholesterol and risks of cardiovascular diseases.

1. Ibid, pp. 317

The presence of an essential amino acids called lysine along with other elements are said to help fight against free radicals that result in aging or the formation of malignant cells.

Bleeding Tendencies

Amaranth is valuable in all kinds of bleeding tendencies. A cupful of fresh leaf juice mixed with a teaspoonful of lime juice is advised every night in conditions such as bleeding from the gums, nose, lungs, piles and excessive menstruation. It is a natural tonic.

ASPARAGUS

Botanical Name: *Asparagus officinalis*
Indian Names: *Shatwār, Soot mooli and Halyan*

Asparagus is cultivated mostly for its tender shoots, commonly known as spears. This vegetable is of importance because of the valuable salts, vitamins and large amount of cellulose it contains. Asparagus is a perennial plant, with underground fleshy root-stock. The young shoots are eaten when 6 to 15 cm high.

Origin and Distribution: Asparagus is a native of the eastern Mediterranean and Asia Minor. Over centuries it has been taken from the wild into cultivated fields and gardens and progressively improved. Several wild species are found in China, the tuberous roots of some of which are used as food and in medicine. Asparagus is now an important crop, especially in Taiwan where the shoots are canned for export. It is widely grown in East Africa and Malaysia.

Natural Benefits and Curative Properties

Asparagus has multiple therapeutic properties. It is an excellent body cleanser. This alkaline vegetable prevents or combats blood acidity. It has a nitrogenous content called 'asparagin' which has diuretic properties. Liberal use of young shoots acts as a rejuvenator.

Asparagus*

Food Value		Minerals and Vitamins	
Moisture	93.0%	Calcium	22 mg
Protein	2.2%	Phosphorus	62 mg
Fat	0.2%	Mangesium	20 mg
Fibre	0.7%	Iron	1.0 mg
Carbohydrates	3.9%	Vitamin A	900 IU**
	100%	Vitamin C	33 mg
		Small amounts of Vit B Complex	

**Values per 100 gms edible portion | Calorific Value - 59 | **Int'l Unit*

However, use of asparagus should be avoided in goitre, liver and kidney diseases and excess mucus, especially catarrh mucus.[1]

Rheumatism

On account of its potash content asparagus is a valuable food medicine in rheumatism. However, it should be steamed and not boiled; with boiling it loses about four-fifth of the valuable salts. An infusion of asparagus is considered highly beneficial in treatment of chronic gout. It should be given in doses of 30 to 60 ml. In advanced stages of kidney diseases[2] it should, however, be avoided.

Heart Disease

Asparagus is an excellent food for strengthening the heart. A food medicine for weak or enlarged hearts is prepared by mixing the freshly expressed juice of this vegetable with honey and taking a teaspoonful three times daily. Patients with heart disease benefit by eating it as a steamed vegetable.

Sexual Debility

In Unani[3] medicine the dried roots of asparagus are used as an aphrodisiac. It is available in market as *Safed musli*. Roots boiled in milk are used as demulcent or soothing medicine. Its regular use thickens semen and is a remedy for impotency.

---

1. Lelord Kordel, *Health the Easy Way*, p.p 131, Award Book, New York, 1976.
2. Dr. S.J. Singh, *Food Remedies* p. 25, Nature Cure Council of Medical Research, Lucknow, 1982.
3. Unani Medicine is a form of traditional medicine practiced in Middle-East and South-Asian countries.

BEET ROOT

Botanical Name: *Beta vulgaris*
Indian Name: *Chukandar*

The red beet, commonly known as garden beet, is a juicy root vegetable distinguished by its unique flavour. Beets have several varieties grouped according to shape. They are flat, short, top-shaped, deep oblate to round, globular to oval, and longish. It is more colourful than other root vegetables. The two varieties most commonly grown in India are Crimson Globe and Detroit Dark Red, both belonging to globular to oval group.

Origin and Distribution: Beet is believed to be a native of the Mediterranean region or of areas around West Asia. It has been used as a vegetable for 2,000 years; even the early Greeks and Romans are known to have used it. It is now widely distributed in the tropics. In India it is cultivated for its nutritious roots.

Food Value: This vegetable is a good tonic food. It contains carbohydrates, mainly in the form of sugar, and some protein and fat. Beet is taken in a variety of ways. It is widely used in salads and in preparing pickles and chutneys. They are also baked like potatoes or boiled, steamed or cooked. It is important to thoroughly wash the vegetable before boiling and to remove the skin before using. The leaves, like all green vegetables, should be cooked with a small amount of water and only for a short time. The fresher the beets, the better the flavour and quicker they cook.

Beet juice is considered as one of the best of all vegetable juices. It is a rich source of natural sugar, as well as contains sodium, potassium, phosphorus, calcium, sulphur, chlorine, iodine, iron, copper, vitamin B_1, B_2, niacin, B_6, C and P. It is also rich in easily digestible carbohydrates but has low calorie content. The protein factors or amino acids are good in both quality and quantity.

Beet Root*

Food Value		Minerals and Vitamins	
Moisture	87.7%	Calcium	18 mg
Protein	1.7%	Phosphorus	55 mg
Fat	0.1%	Iron	1.0 mg
Minerals	0.8%	Vitamin C	10 mg
Fibre	0.9%	Good amounts of Vit A & B and small amount of Vit B Complex	
Carbohydrates	8.8%		
	100%		

**Values per 100 gms edible portion | Calorific Value - 43*

Natural Benefits and Curative Properties

Beets are of great therapeutic value. They have properties to cleanse the kidneys and gall bladder. Being rich in alkaline elements, potassium, calcium, magnesium and iron, they are useful in combating acidosis and aid the natural processes of elimination.

Anaemia

Red beet juice is associated with blood forming qualities. Due to its higher content of iron, it regenerates and reactivates the red blood cells, supplies fresh oxygen to the body and helps in normal functioning of vesicular breathing i.e. normal breath sound. It is thus extremely useful in the treatment of anaemia.

According to Dr. Fritz Keitel of Germany, 'The juice of red beet strengthens the body's powers of resistance and has proved to be an excellent remedy for anaemia, especially for children and teenagers where other blood forming remedies have failed.'[1]

Digestive Disorders

Beet juice is beneficial in treating jaundice, hepatitis, nausea and vomiting due to biliousness, diarrhoea and dysentery. Adding a teaspoonful of lime juice increases its medicinal value and can be given as a liquid food. Fresh beet juice mixed with a tablespoonful of honey taken every morning before breakfast helps in healing gastric ulcer.[2]

1. Linda Clark, *Handbook of Natural Remedies for Common Ailments*, pp. 44, Pocket Books, New York, 1976.
2. N.W. Walker, *Raw Vegetable Juices*, pp. 34, Jove Books, New York, 1983.

Leaves of beet root eaten as green-leafy vegetable and its juice, mixed with lime juice, are both valuable in hepatitis or jaundice and gastric ulcer. The juice should be taken once daily.

Constipation

Cellulose content of the beet acts as a bulk residue, increases peristalsis i.e. wavelike movement which ease the passage of stool. Its regular use prevents habitual constipation. A decoction of the beet root is highly valuable in chronic constipation and haemorrhoids. It may be given in doses of half to one small glass at bed time.

Circulatory Disorders

Beet juice is an excellent solvent for inorganic calcium deposits. It is valuable in treatment of hypertension, arteriosclerosis, heart trouble and varicose veins.

Kidney and Gall Bladder Disorders

Beet juice, in combination with the juice of carrot and cucumber, is one of the finest natural cleansing agents for kidneys and gall bladder. It is highly beneficial in all disorders of these two organs.

Skin Disorders

The water in which beet roots and tops have been boiled make an excellent application for boils, skin inflammation and pimples and pustules. White beet is better for this purpose. For an irritable skin the body should be sponged occasionally with a mixture of three parts of beet water to one part of white vinegar. This mixture is also useful as a skin wash in cases of measles and eruptive fevers.

Dandruff

The decoction of beets mixed with a little vinegar can be used before bath to cleanse or scurf the dandruff. Beet water can also be massaged into the scalp with the ginger tip every night.

BITTER GOURD

Botanical Name: *Monordica charantia*
Indian Name: *Karelā*

Bitter gourd is a common vegetable cultivated extensively in India. It is 10 to 20 cm long, tapering at the ends and covered with blunt tubercles. The seeds are white in raw fruits and become red when ripe. Bitter gourd has two varieties. One is long, oblong and pale green in colour. The other is small, little oval and dark green. Both are bitter in taste. They turn reddish-orange when ripe.

Origin and Distribution: The original home of bitter gourd is not known except that it is a native of the tropics. It is widely grown in India, Indonesia, Sri Lanka, Malayasia, the Philippines, China and the Caribbean.

Bitter Gourd*

Food Value		Minerals and Vitamins	
Moisture	92.4%	Calcium	20 mg
Protein	1.6%	Phosphorus	70 mg
Fat	0.2%	Iron	1.8 mg
Minerals	0.8%	Vitamin C	88 mg
Fibre	0.8%	Small amounts of Vitamin B Complex	
Carbohydrates	4.2%		
	100%		

**Values per 100 gms edible portion | Calorific Value - 25*

Natural Benefits and Curative Properties

Bitter gourd has excellent medicinal properties. It is antidotal, antipyretic tonic, appetizing, stomachic, anti-bilious and a laxative[1]. It is also used in traditional medicines of Asia and Africa.

Diabetes

Bitter gourd has been used as a specific folk medicine for diabetes. Recent researches by British doctors have established that it contains

1. J.F. Dastur, *Medicinal Plants of India and Pakistan*, pp. 112, D.B. Taraporevala Sons & Co. (P) Ltd., Bombay, 1985.

a hypoglycaemic or insulin-like principle, designated as 'plant-insulin', which has been found highly beneficial in lowering blood and urine sugar levels. It should, therefore, be included liberally in the diabetic diet. For better results, juice of about four or five fruits every morning on empty stomach is recommended. The seeds of bitter gourd can be added to the food in powdered form. Diabetics can also use bitter gourd decoction prepared by boiling cut pieces in water or by dissolving dry powder of seeds in water.

A majority of diabetics are usually under-nourished. Bitter gourd being rich in all essential vitamins and minerals, especially vitamin A, B_1, B_2, C and Iron, its regular use prevents complications associated with diabetes such as hypertension, eye complications, neuritis and defective metabolism of carbohydrates. It strengthens immunity against infection.

Piles

Juice of the fresh leaves of bitter gourd is valuable in piles. Three teaspoonfuls of the juice mixed in a glassful of buttermilk is advised every morning for about a month. A paste of roots of bitter gourd plant can also be applied over piles with beneficial results.

Blood Disorders

Bitter gourd is highly beneficial in treating blood disorders like blood boils, scabies, itching, psoriasis, ring-worm and other fungal diseases. A cupful of fresh juice of bitter gourd mixed with a teaspoonful of lime juice should be sipped slowly on empty stomach daily for four to six months in these conditions. Its regular use in endemic regions of leprosy acts as a preventive medicine.[1]

Respiratory Disorders

Bitter gourd plant roots have been used in folk medicine for respiratory disorders since the ancient times. A teaspoonful of root paste mixed with an equal amount of honey or *tulsi* leaf juice, given once every night for a month makes for an excellent remedy for asthma, bronchitis, pharyngitis, colds and rhinitis.

---

1. S.A. Majeed. *Tibbe-Rahamani*, Urdu, pp. 118, 1928.

Alcoholism

Leaf juice is an antidote for alcohol intoxication. It is also useful in liver damage resulting from alcoholism.

Cholera

Fresh juice of leaves of bitter gourd is an effective medicine in early stages of cholera and other types of diarrhoea during summer. Two teaspoonfuls of juice mixed with equal quantity of white onion juice and a teaspoonful of lime juice is advised.

Uses

Bitter gourd is eaten as a cooked vegetable in India and the Far East. The bitterness is reduced by steeping the peeled fruit in salt water solution before cooking. It is also used in pickles and as an ingredient in curries. The seeds of the ripe fruit are used as a condiment. The tender shoots and leaves are used as spinach.

BOTTLE GOURD

Botanical Name: *Lagenaria vulgaris*
Indian Names: *Lauki, Doodhi and Ghia*

Bottle gourd is a common vegetable. It is yellowish green, having the shape of a bottle with white pulp and white seeds embedded in spongy flesh.

Origin and Distribution: Bottle gourd is amongst the earliest vegetables cultivated by man. It is a warm season crop which grows best in a warm humid climate. It appears to have originated in Africa or India where it occurs spontaneously. It is now widely cultivated throughout the tropics, especially India, Indonesia, Malaysia, Philippines, China, tropical Africa and South America.

Natural Benefits and Curative Properties

The cooked vegetable is cooling, diuretic, sedative and anti-bilious. Eating bottle gourd gives a feeling of relaxation. However, it should not be eaten raw as it may prove harmful for stomach and intestines.

Bottle Gourd*

Food Value		Minerals and Vitamins	
Moisture	96.1%	Calcium	20 mg
Protein	0.2%	Phosphorus	10 mg
Fat	0.1%	Iron	0.7 mg
Minerals	0.5%	Small amounts of Vitamin B Complex	
Fibre	0.6%		
Carbohydrates	2.5%		
	100%		

**Values per 100 gms edible portion | Calorific Value - 12*

Urinary Disorders

Bottle gourd is valuable in urinary disorders. Due to its alkaline nature a glassful of fresh juice prepared by grating the whole fruit mixed with teaspoonful of lime juice is given once daily to treat burning sensation in the urinary passage resulting from high acidity of urine. In treating urinary infection it should be given with sulpha drugs. It acts as an alkaline diuretic.

Excessive Thirst

Juice of bottle gourd is a valuable medicine for excessive thirst due to severe diarrhoea, diabetes and excessive use of fatty or fried foods. A glassful of plain juice with a pinch of salt should be taken everyday. During summer it prevents excessive loss of sodium, quenches thirst and helps in preventing fatigue.

Insomnia

Mixture of bottle gourd juice and sesame oil massaged over the scalp every night acts as an effective medicine for insomnia.

CABBAGE

Botanical Names: *Brassica oleracea var, capitala*
Indian Names: *Bandgobhi, Karam kalla and Pattagobhi*

Cabbage is one of the most highly rated leafy-vegetables. It is grown for its large, edible, terminal buds and eaten the world over. There are several varieties differing in size, shape and colour of leaves, and texture of the head. Cabbage is an excellent muscle builder and a cleanser.

Origin and Distribution: Cabbage was cultivated long before the dawn of recorded history. The ancient Greeks and the Roman considered it an important vegetable. The original home of cabbage are the Mediterranean regions. The major areas of cultivation now are North India, Indonesia, Malaysia, the Philippines, Central, East and West Africa, Central and South America and the Caribbean.

Food Value: Cabbage is primarily valued for its high mineral and vitamin content and alkaline salts. It can be used raw in salads, or steamed, boiled and cooked. For best results it should be eaten raw; valuable nutrients are mostly lost in cooking. Raw cabbage is also more easily digested. The longer the cabbage is cooked, the less digestible it becomes. It can be rectified by adding some asafoetida i.e. *hing*. The cabbage with green leaves is especially valuable because of high content of vitamin A.

Natural Benefits and Curative Properties

Cabbage has wonderful cleansing and reducing properties. Its most valuable properties are the high sulphur and chlorine content and a relatively large percentage of iodine. The combination of sulphur and chlorine cleanse the mucus membranes of the stomach and intestinal tract but only when cabbage or its juice is taken raw without salt.

However, cabbage and its juice should never be taken as main part of the diet. Excessive intake has been known to cause goitre, a thyroid disease. It is only in normal helpings that cabbage is

Cabbage*

Food Value		Minerals and Vitamins	
Moisture	91.9%	Calcium	39 mg
Protein	1.8%	Phosphorus	44 mg
Fat	0.1%	Iron	0.8 mg
Minerals	0.6%	Vitamin C	124 mg
Fibre	1.0%	Small amounts of	
Carbohydrates	4.6%	Vitamin B Complex	
	100%		

**Values per 100 gms edible portion | Calorific Value - 27*

nutritionally valuable. Its juice, which is bitter and not particularly delicious, constitutes an important part of natural regime to cure infections, ulcers and other disorders of the digestive system.[1]

Constipation

Cabbage provides roughage essential to stimulate proper bowel action. A meal of raw cabbage is an excellent remedy for constipation. It acts quickly without any adverse after-effects. This meal can be prepared by adding a little salt, black pepper and lemon juice to finely chopped raw cabbage.

Stomach Ulcers

Duodenal ulcers have responded almost miraculously to cabbage juice. Its origin as a traditional remedy goes back to the work of Garnet Cheney, M.D. of Stanford University School of Medicine

> Your diet is a bank account.
> Good food choices are good investments.
> Bethenny Frankel, Philanthropist

some forty years ago. He is reported to have cured many ulcer patients with raw cabbage juice. The juice contains an anti-ulcer factor, vitamin U which is destroyed by cooking. The treatment consists of taking 90 to 180 gm of cabbage juice three times daily followed by a natural diet.

To make the juice palatable Dr. Cheney often added celery juice of stalk and greens, pineapple juice, tomato juice or a citrus juice. Chilling the mixed juice also helps to improve the flavour. The juice, however, should be taken with several intervals throughout the day and never in one go. If one does not have a juicer or a blender, one can nibble on raw cabbage four or five times a day.[2]

1. Susane E. Charmine, *The Complete Raw Juice Therapy*, pp. 59, Thorsons Publishing Group, Great Britain, 1987.
2. Mark Bricklin, *Rodale's Encyclopedia of Natural Home Remedies*, p. 466, D.B. Taraporevala Son and Co (P) Lid, Bombay, 1982.

Obesity

Recent research has discovered a valuable content called tartronic acid in cabbage which inhibits conversion of sugar and other carbohydrates into fat. It is therefore of great value in weight reduction. Eating cabbage salad is one of the simplest methods of dieting and staying slim.

A hundred grams of cabbage has only 27 kilocalories of energy while the same quantity of wheat bread will yield about 240 calories. Cabbage has been found to possess maximum biological value with minimum calorific value. Moreover, it gives a lasting feeling of fullness in the stomach and is easily digestible.

Skin Disorders

Cabbage leaves have been successfully used as compresses in healing ulcers, infected sores, blisters and skin eruptions, including psoriasis. They are also valuable in burns and carbuncles. The thickest and greenest outer leaves are most effective as compress. The whole leaf should be used for a large compress.

After removing the thick veins cabbage leaves should be flattened, made soft and smooth by rolling them with a rolling pin. They should be warmed, dried with a towel and then applied smoothly to the affected part in an overlapping manner. The leaves may be cut into thin strips for treating a small area. The cabbage leaves should be placed on a linen cloth and a pad of soft woollen cloth put over it. The whole compress should then be secured with an elastic bandage. The compress can be kept for the full duration of one day and night. If, however, the leaves wither or change colour, they should be replaced with fresh ones. Before changing the compress, affected area should be thoroughly washed and dried.[1]

Premature Ageing

Research has shown that cabbage contains several elements and properties which enhance immunity and arrest premature ageing. The vegetable is of great value for persons of advancing age. Some

1. Dr. S.J. Singh, *Food Remedies*, pp. 52-53, Nature Cure Council of Medical Research, Lucknow, 1982.

of its properties help prevent formation of patches on the walls of blood vessels and stones in the gall bladder. A combination of vitamin P and C in cabbage strengthens blood vessels.

CARROT

Botanical Name: *Daucus carota*
Indian Name: *Gājar*

Carrot is a popular vegetable. It is a powerful cleansing food. Green carrot leaves are highly nutritive, rich in protein, minerals and vitamins.

Broadly, carrot can be classified into two groups, namely, the Asiatic type and the European type. The former is larger size, darker colour and sweet taste. However, the latter are preferred due to their smooth surface, thin core and being less fibrous.

Origin and Distribution: Carrot probably originated in Central Asia, in the hills of Punjab and Kashmir in India, with secondary centres of distribution in Asia, Europe and Mediterranean North Africa. It is cultivated in India, Malaysia, Indonesia, Philippines, Central, East and West Africa, South America and the Caribbean.

Food Value: Carrot is an extremely rich source of vitamin A. The name carotene, which is a form of pro-vitamin, has been derived from carrot. Carotene is converted to vitamin A by the liver and stored in the body.

Carrots are rich in sodium, sulphur, chlorine and contain traces of iodine. The mineral content in carrots lie very close to the skin, hence peeling or scraping should be avoided.

Natural Benefits and Curative Properties

Carrots are rich in alkaline elements which purify and revitalise the blood. It nourishes the entire system and help in maintaining acid-alkaline balance in the body.

Carrot*

Food Value		Minerals and Vitamins	
Moisture	86.0%	Calcium	80 mg
Protein	0.9%	Phosphorus	530 mg
Fat	0.2%	Iron	2.2 mg
Minerals	1.1%	Vitamin C	3 mg
Fibre	1.2%	Small amounts of	
Carbohydrates	10.6%	Vitamin B Complex	
	100%		

**Values per 100 gms edible portion | Calorific Value - 48*

Carrot juice is called a "miracle juice". It makes a fine health-giving drink for children and adults alike. It strengthens the eyes and keeps the mucus membranes of all cavities of the body in healthy condition. It is beneficial in the treatment of dry and rough skin.

Use of carrot seeds should be avoided during early pregnancy as these can increase the toxicity of uterine walls and cause abortion.

Tooth Decay

Chewing a carrot immediately after food kills all harmful germs in the mouth. It cleanses the teeth, removes food particles lodged in the crevices and prevents bleeding gums and tooth decay.

Digestive Disorders

Chewing carrots increases saliva and speeds up digestion by supplying enzymes, minerals and vitamins necessary for digestion. Regular use of carrot prevents the formation of gastric ulcer and other digestive disorders. Carrot juice is an effective remedy in ailments like intestinal colic, colitis, appendicitis, peptic ulcer and dyspepsia.

Constipation

Carrot juice, combined with spinach juice and a little lemon juice, is very effective in treating constipation. Spinach juice cleanses the bowels. The full effect takes about two months and the bowel movement becomes regular. About 50 ml of spinach juice should be added to 250 ml of carrot juice to make this combination.

Diarrhoea

Carrot soup is an effective natural remedy for diarrhoea. It supplies fluid to combat dehydration, replenishes sodium, potassium, phosphorus, calcium, sulphur and magnesium. It is a good source of pectin and coats the intestines which prevents inflammation. It also checks the growth of harmful bacteria and prevents vomiting, especially in children. About half a kilogram of carrot may be cooked in 150 ml of water until soft. The pulp should be strained, salt added to taste and a small amount of the soup given to the patient every half an hour. Improvement is usually noticeable in about 24 hours.[1]

Thread Worms

Carrots are offensive to all parasites and valuable in eliminating thread worms in children. A small cupful of grated carrot taken every morning, with no other food added to the meal, can clear worms and other parasites quickly.

Fertility

Raw carrots are good for fertility. Sterility can sometimes be overcome by consuming raw carrots. The cause of sterility has been traced to the continuous use of food in which enzymes are destroyed by cooking or pasteurizing.

Uses

Carrots can be used in a variety of ways, in raw salads, or boiled or cooked. They can also be used in soups and juice. They are most useful when taken raw. In cooking, a large amount of the important minerals are lost.

---

1. Linda Clark, *Handbook of Natural Remedies for Common Ailments*, p. 131, Pocket Books, New York, 1977.

CUCUMBER

Botanical Name: *Cucumis sativas*
Indian Name: *Kheeā*

Cucumber is a popular, widely cultivated vegetable. It has a cooling and refreshing effect. It contains almost all essential elements needed for preserving health.

There are several varieties of cucumber differing in shape, size and colour, with colour varying from whitish green to dark green. The colour turns orange or brownish yellow when cucumber matures. Its size ranges from 8 to 30 cm or more. The best variety for use is fresh, firm, smooth, regular in shape and dark green in colour.

Origin and Distribution: Cucumber is believed to have originated in northern India. It was known to ancient Egyptians, Greeks and Romans and available in China by the sixth century AD. The main areas of cultivation today include India, South East Asia, Africa, Central and South America, the Caribbean and most tropical areas.

Food Value: Cucumber has a high mineral content. It should not be peeled; the skin is very valuable as the cell salts and vitamins are in and near it.

Cucumber is a valuable source of potassium, sodium, magnesium, sulphur, silicon, chlorine and fluorine. It is generally used as a salad in combination with carrot, beet, tomato, radish, lettuce and other vegetables. Adding some curd to the salad makes it tastier and adds to nutritional value.

Cucumber*

Food Value		**Minerals and Vitamins**	
Moisture	96.3%	Calcium	10 mg
Protein	0.4%	Phosphorus	25 mg
Fat	0.1%	Iron	1.5 mg
Minerals	0.3%	Vitamin C	7 mg
Fibre	0.4%	Small amounts of	
Carbohydrates	2.5%	Vitamin B Complex	
	100%		

**Values per 100 gms edible portion | Calorific Value - 13*

Natural Benefits and Curative Properties

Cucumber has 64 per cent alkaline-forming minerals and 36 per cent acid forming minerals which make it rich in remedial and curative properties especially useful in maintaining alkalinity of the blood. It is also one of the best natural diuretics. It should always be taken raw; potassium and phosphorus are lost in cooking.

Constipation

Cucumber is a dependable laxative food. It supplies bulk to aid the bowel action. Those who suffer from constipation benefit greatly by taking two cucumbers a day.

Stomach Disorders

Juice of cucumber is a valuable food medicine in the treatment of hyperacidity, gastric and duodenal ulcers. It should be taken in doses of four to six tablespoons every two hours in such conditions. Sufficient juice can be extracted from a cucumber; 96 per cent of cucumber is water. Juice gives immediate relief in case of burning sensation in the stomach.

Rheumatism/Rheumatic Ailments

Cucumber juice in combination with the juice of carrots, beets and celery has a beneficial effect in conditions associated with accumulation of uric acid such as arthritis, gout and rheumatism.

Urinary Disorders

Cucumber seeds are rich in potassium. Emulsion of shelled seeds has been found highly beneficial in treating burning sensation in urinary calculi or stone in individuals predisposed to such disorders. This emulsion mixed with curd is useful in dissolving the gravel in the urinary tract and reducing hyperacidity of the urine.[1]

Cholera

A glassful of fresh leaf juice mixed with tender coconut water given one or about 30 ml every hour relieves excessive thirst during cholera. It acts by restoring the electrolyte balance in case of dehydration.

---

1. Dr. Aman, *Medicinal Secrets of Your Food*, pp. 426, Indo American Hospital, Mysore, 1985

Skin Eruptions

Cucumber juice has proved effective in cases of skin eruption; juices of carrot and lettuce can be added for better results. In some cases addition of a little alfalfa juice helps to make it more efficacious.

Beauty Aid

Grated cucumber applied over face, eyes and neck for 15 to 20 minutes is an effective beauty aid and a good tonic for the facial skin. Its regular use prevents pimples, blackheads, wrinkles and dryness of the face. Due to its high silicon and sulphur content cucumber juice promotes hair growth particularly when mixed with carrot, lettuce and spinach juice.

DRUMSTICK

Botanical Name: *Moringa oleifera*
Indian Name: *Sanjanā*

Drumstick is a fairly common vegetable grown in the Indian sub-continent. It is valued mainly for its tender pod which is antibacterial and a wonderful cleanser.

Drumstick is a perennial, erect, slender, medium sized tree with arching branches. It has a drumstick like fruit, small white flowers and round leaves which are cooked and eaten as a vegetable. It is also grown in backyards of South Indian homes.

Food Value: Drumstick pods and leaves are a great source of carotene, calcium, phosphorus and vitamin C. The leaves, flowers and fruits of drumstick used as vegetable and have high nutritional value. The tender fruit is used in most South Indian dishes, including *sambar*. The leaves and flowers are used to prepare curry and cake.

Natural Benefits and Curative Properties

Almost all parts of the drumstick tree have therapeutic value. The leaves have medicinal properties and are rich in iron.

Drumstick (Pods)*

Food Value		Minerals and Vitamins	
Moisture	86.9%	Calcium	30 mg
Protein	2.5%	Phosphorus	110 mg
Fat	0.1%	Iron	5.3 mg
Minerals	2.0%	Vitamin C	120 mg
Fibre	4.8%	Small amounts of	
Carbohydrates	3.7%	Vitamin B Complex	
	100%		

Calorific Value - 26

Drumstick (Leaves)*

Food Value		Minerals and Vitamins	
Moisture	75.9%	Calcium	440 mg
Protein	6.7%	Phosphorus	70 mg
Fat	1.7%	Iron	7 mg
Minerals	2.3%	Vitamin C	220 mg
Fibre	0.9%	Small amounts of	
Carbohydrates	12.5%	Vitamin B Complex	
	100%		

**Values per 100 gms edible portion | Calorific Value - 92*

Tonic for Children

The leaves serve as a tonic for infants and growing children. Juice extracted from leaves filtered and mixed with milk is an excellent tonic for healthy and strong bones and for purifying blood.

Pregnancy and Lactation

The above tonic taken regularly provides expectant mothers with necessary calcium, iron and vitamins. It facilitates easy delivery and reduces post delivery complications. A vegetable prepared by boiling the leaves with salt and water and smearing the leaves with ghee after draining the water increases secretion of breast milk.

Respiratory Disorder

A soup of drumstick leaves is highly beneficial in treating respiratory diseases like asthma, bronchitis and tuberculosis. The soup is prepared by adding a handful of leaves to 180 ml of water and boiling for five minutes. A little salt, pepper and lime juice may be added to enhance taste.[1]

1. Dr. Aman, *Medicinal Secrets of Your Food*, pp. 341, Indo-American Hospital, Mysore, 1985.

Infections

Drumstick soup made by boiling the leaves, flowers and drumsticks is valuable in preventing infections of the throat, chest and skin. This is due to the antibacterial properties of the drumstick which are much like penicillin and other antibiotics.

Sexual Disorders

A soup made with drumstick flowers boiled in milk acts as a useful sex tonic. It is also useful in functional sterility in both males and females.

The powder of the dry bark is valuable in impotency, premature ejaculation and thin semen. An infusion of 120 gm of powder of dry bark boiled for half an hour in 600 ml of water given in doses of 30 ml with a table spoonful of honey three times daily for a month to cure these conditions.[1]

Digestive Disorders

Drumstick is valuable in treating digestive disorders. A teaspoonful of fresh leaf juice, mixed with honey and a glassful of tender coconut water is given two or three times a day in treatment of cholera, dysentery, diarrhoea, colitis and hepatitis or jaundice.

Urinary Disorders

A tablespoonful of coagulated fresh leaf juice, mixed with a glass of fresh juice of cucumber or carrot is an effective medicine for scanty urination and constant burning in urethra caused by high acidity of urine. A teaspoonful of the juice with 10 gm of rock-salt once a day, is used to cure excessive urination of non-diabetics.[2]

Beauty-Aid

Fresh leaf juice applied with lime juice is useful in the treatment of pimples and black heads and to keep the face skin looking fresh.

---

1. Ibid., pp. 343-344.
2. Ibid., pp. 342.

FENUGREEK

Botanical Name: *Trigonella foenum-graecum*
Indian Name: *Methi*

Fenugreek is a well-known leafy vegetable with rich medicinal virtues. It is nature's great boon to mankind and its regular use helps keep the body healthy. It has been used since the ancient times both as a food and as a medicine by people along living on the Mediterranean and in Asia.

Fenugreek is an erect, strongly scented, robust, annual herb, about 30 to 60 cm high. It has compound leaves of light green colour 2 to 2.5 cm long, auxiliary yellow flowers, and thin pointed pods. The seeds are brownish yellow and emit a peculiar odour.

There are two popular varieties of fenugreek known as *Masuri Methi* or *Champa Methi,* and *Marwari Methi.* Both varieties are scented and are recommended for cultivation.

Origin and Distribution: Fenugreek is considered to be a native of eastern Europe and Ethopia. It is a cool season crop and grows throughout India.

Food Value: In India, the plants and leaves of fenugreek are commonly used as a culinary vegetable known as *methi-ka-saag.* Steaming is the best method of cooking fenugreek leaves; this retains the vitamins and makes the vegetable tastier. The dried leaves are comparable to pulses for their protein content. They supplement the lysine-deficient cereal diets; lysine is an amino acid and a fundamental constituent of all proteins. The seeds of fenugreek contain a foetid and biller fatty oil resin, mucilage and albumin. Their mineral and vitamin contents are very high. In Indian homes, seeds are generally used as a condiment for flavouring.

Natural Benefits and Curative Properties

The leaves of fenugreek are aromatic, cooling and mildly aperient. Paste of the fresh leaves applied regularly before bathing on the scalp, lengthens hair, preserves natural colour and keeps the hair

Fenugreek*

Food Value		Minerals and Vitamins	
Moisture	86.1%	Calcium	395 mg
Protein	4.4%	Phosphorus	51 mg
Fat	0.9%	Iron	16.5 mg
Minerals	1.5%	Vitamin C	52 mg
Fibre	1.1%	Small amounts of Vitamin B Complex	
Carbohydrates	6.0%		
	100%		

**Values per 100 gms edible portion | Calorific Value - 49*

silky soft. Paste of fresh leaves applied on the face every night before bedtime and washed with warm water, prevents pimples, blackheads, dryness and early appearance of wrinkles. It improves complexion and makes one look younger. Seeds of fenugreek are demulcent, diuretic, carminative (relieve gastric discomfort), galactagogue, (increases the flow of milk), astringent and an aphrodisiac tonic.[1] They are the best cleansers of body, highly mucus-solvents and soothing agents. The seeds are used in the preparation of hair tonics and cosmetics in some parts of the world.

Digestive Disorders

Fenugreek leaves are highly beneficial in treating indigestion, flatulence and sluggish liver. An infusion of the leaves used as a gargle helps heal recurrent mouth ulcers. Boiled and fried in butter, they are valuable in biliousness. The seeds are also useful in the treatment of colic, flatulence, dysentery, diarrhoea and dyspepsia.

Anaemia

The leaves help in blood formation. Cooked fenugreek leaves help prevent anaemic condition generally associated with the onset of puberty and sudden spurt of growth especially of adoloscent girls. Being rich in iron, fenugreek seeds are valuable in curing anaemia.

Pregnancy and Lactation

A preparation of finely powdered seeds fried in ghee helps in quick normalisation after delivery. The powder is mixed with wheat flour

1. J.F. Dastur, *Medicinal Plants of India and Pakistan*, pp. 169, D.B. Taraporevala Sons & Co. (P) Ltd., Bombay, 1985.

and sugar to prepare a *halwa* which is eaten in small quantities daily. The seeds, made into a gruel, are given as a diet to nursing mothers for increasing the flow of milk.

Deadened Sense of Taste and Smell

The seeds help restore deadened sense of taste and smell. The taste loss occurs due to improper functioning of the salivary glands; they often become plugged with mucus and accumulated juices causing swelling. Similarly, the sense of smell can get obstructed by long accumulations of mucus or other impurities in the nose where olfactory nerves are based. Regular use of fenugreek is beneficial in both cases.

Dandruff

Fenugreek seeds are useful in getting rid of dandruff. Two tablespoonfuls of the seeds are soaked overnight in water and the softened seeds ground into a fine paste the next morning which is applied over the scalp and left for half an hour. The hair is then washed thoroughly with soap nut solution (or *shikakai*) to cure dandruff. A paste of the fresh leaves of fenugreek applied over the scalp regularly before taking bath also cures dandruff.

Fevers

A tea made from fenugreek seeds is equal in value to quinine for reducing fevers. It is particularly valuable as a cleansing and soothing drink. Fenugreek seeds, when moistened with water are themselves slightly mucilageous. A tea made from them has the power to dissolve even the more sticky substance as the body mucus.

Stomach Disorders

Fenugreek tea soothes inflamed stomach and intestines, and cleanses stomach, bowels, kidneys and respiratory tract of excess mucus. It is also beneficial in healing peptic ulcers. The mild coating of gum like lubricant material deposited by fenugreek while passing through the stomach and intestines provides a protective shell for the ulcers.[1]

---

1. Lelord Kordel, *Health The Easy Way*, pp. 48, Award Books, New York, 1976.

Respiratory Infections

During early acute stages of any of the respiratory tract infections such as bronchitis, influenza, sinusitis, catarrh and suspected pneumonia, fenugreek tea helps the body to prespire, dispel toxicity and shorten the period of fever. Four cups the tea should be taken daily. The quantity is reduced as the condition improves. For flavour a few drops of lemon juice can be added. Fasting has to be observed during the treatment (no other form of food or nourishment should be taken) to allow the body to correct these respiratory problems in a few days.

Sore Throat

The gargle made from fenugreek seeds is the best remedy for ordinary sore throat. The gargle solution should be much stronger than fenugreek tea. Two tablespoonfuls of fenugreek seeds are soaked in about 1 litre of cold water and allowed to simmer for half an hour over a low flame. The solution is then cooled to a bearable temperature, strained and the entire quantity used as a gargle.

Bad breath and Body Odour

Tea made from fenugreek is also beneficial in cases of bad breath and body odour. Unpleasant odours emanate from the body openings due to accumulations of hardened mucus and other toxic substances in the nasal and oral passages, the gastrointestinal tract, the urinary tract, the bloodstream and the vagina. Fenugreek tea taken regularly helps remove these accumulations from spots where mouth wash and soap can never penetrate.

Diabetes

Fenugreek seeds have been found highly effective in the treatment of diabetes. According to a report published by the Indian Council of Medical Research quoted by Press Trust of India on January 6, 1988, fenugreek seeds given in varying doses of 25 gms to 100 gms daily, diminish reactive hyperglycaemia in diabetic patients. Levels of glucose, serum cholesterol and triglycerides were also significantly reduced in diabetes patients when the seeds were consumed, the report said quoting researchers at the National

Institute of Nutrition, Hyderabad. The report further said that the effect of taking fenugreek seeds could be quite dramatic when consumed with 1200-1400 calories diet per day, which is usually recommended for diabetic patients.

Swellings
Due to their cooling properties, a poultice of the leaves can be applied with advantage in external and internal swellings and burns.

GARLIC

Botanical Name: *Allium sativum*
Indian Name: *Lahasoon*

Garlic is a garden vegetable of the onion family. It has been variously described as a food, a herb, a medicinal plant, an antiseptic, a beauty accessory and a magical antidote to evil.

Garlic is an important condiment crop. It is an erect biennial herb normally grown annually. The bulb consists of 6 to 35 bulblets called cloves wrapped in a thin whitish, transparent covering.

Origin and Distribution: Garlic is believed to have originated in Central Asia and was known to the Chinese as early as 3,000 BC. In ancient China, India Egypt, Greece and Rome garlic was used both as a staple food and a medicine.

An analysis of garlic shows it to contain a high percentage of minerals and vitamins with traces of iodine, sulphur and chlorine.

Natural Benefits and Curative Properties

Food Value: For centuries garlic has been held in high esteem for its health qualities. Khnoum Khoufouf, the builder of one of the oldest pyramids, circa 4500 BC, was among the first to recognise virtues of garlic and decreed that all his workers take garlic every day to maintain health and strength.

Garlic*

Food Value		Minerals and Vitamins	
Moisture	62.0%	Calcium	30 mg
Protein	6.3%	Phosphorus	310 mg
Fat	0.1%	Iron	1.3 mg
Minerals	1.0%	Vitamin C	13 mg
Fibre	0.8%	Small amounts of	
Carbohydrates	29.8%	Vitamin B Complex	
	100%		

**Values per 100 gms edible portion | Calorific Value - 145*

Hippocrates, the father of modern medicine (460-357 BC), recommended the use of garlic in infectious diseases and prescribed it especially in intestinal disorders.

In herbal medicine garlic has been traditionally used to treat asthma, deafness, leprosy, bronchial congestion, arteriosclerosis, fevers, worms and liver and gall bladder problems. Babhet, an eminent Ayurvedic authority of ancient India is of the opinion that garlic is good for the heart, is a strengthening food, useful in leucoderma, leprosy, piles, worms, catarrhal disorders, asthma, cough, for hair and as an appetite stimulant.

Recent clinical experiments have confirmed several ancient ideas about healing properties of garlic. These experiments have revealed many more benefits than known previously. The unpleasant odour in garlic is due to its sulphur content. This mineral is largely in its volatile oil which has marvellous therapeutic properties.

With its multiple positive properties garlic helps remove toxins, revitalises blood, stimulates circulation and normalises the intestinal flora. The ethers in the juice are so potent that they dissolve any accumulated mucus in the sinus cavities, the bronchial tubes and the lungs.

Chest Diseases

In treatment of some chest diseases garlic is highly effective. It reduces fetidly of the breath in pulmonary gangrene. Regular use of garlic in tuberculosis of the lungs was advocated by Dr. McDuffie. Dr. F.W. Crosman once said given in sufficient quantities, garlic was a marvellous remedy in treating pneumonia. He used garlic for many years to treat pneumonia. Garlic is also an irritant and rubefacient[1] and can be applied externally on the chest with beneficial results.

In *Ayurveda,* a decoction prepared by boiling one gram of garlic in 240 ml of milk and one litre of water till only one fourth of the decoction remains is advised thrice a day as a highly effective remedy for tuberculosis.

Asthma

Taking three cloves of garlic boiled in milk is recommended in asthma. A pod of garlic peeled and macerated is boiled in 120 ml of pure malt-vinegar. After cooling it is strained and an equal quantity of honey is mixed and the mixture preserved in a clean bottle. One or two teaspoons of this syrup taken with fenugreek decoction at night before retiring has been found effective in reducing the severity of asthmatic attacks.[2]

Digestive Disorders

Garlic has a beneficial effect on the lymph and aids in eliminating the noxious waste matter. It stimulates peristaltic action and the secretion of digestive juices. Crushed cloves of garlic may be infused in water or milk and taken for all types of digestive disorders. It has an antiseptic effect and is an excellent remedy for infectious diseases and any inflammation of the stomach and intestines. The oil of garlic is absorbed into the alimentary tract and is partly eliminated through urine.

Garlic is an excellent worm expeller. It also has a soothing effect in diarrhoea. Problems such as colitis, dysentery and many other intestinal upsets can be successfully treated with fresh garlic. One garlic clove taken three times a day is usually sufficient to correct mild cases of diarrhoea or dysentery. Garlic destroys harmful

---

1. Ibid. pp. 87.
2. Dr. Aman, *Medicinal Secrets of Your Food,* pp. 600 Indo-American Hospital, Mysore, 1985

bacteria in the intestines without affecting the beneficial organisms which aid digestion.

High Blood Pressure/Hypertension

Garlic is regarded as one of the most effective remedies for lowering blood pressure. It also slows the pulse and modifies heart rhythm, besides relieving symptoms of dizziness, shortness of breath and formation of gas in the digestive track. An average dosage of two to three garlic cloves a day is sufficient to dent blood pressure.

Dr. F.G. Piotrowski, University of Geneva, says that garlic has a dilatory effect on the blood vessels, thereby reducing the pressure.

Rheumatism/Rheumatic Afflictions

In Russia garlic is used extensively in treating rheumatism and associated diseases. Garlic is also recommended to rheumatic sufferers in the UK. Recent experiments in Japan tested a garlic extract on patients with lumbago and arthritis and a large number of them benefited without any side-effects. Garlic has been known to exhibit an anti-inflammatory property which could account for its effectiveness in treating arthritis and rheumatism.

Garlic: Nature's Powerful Antibiotic

Garlic can treat or prevent many diseases caused from infection by bacteria, viruses, molds or parasites. For treating cold, flu, bronchitis, dysentery, ulcer other infectious disease, the garlic form used should have antibiotic properties. Not all forms do.

The most important antibiotic constituent in garlic is allicin; some garlic products retain allicin and could theoretically have antibiotic effects, but none can compare to the power, simplicity and economy of taking raw garlic.

Allicin is produced as soon as garlic is cut or chopped, but degrades quickly into a large number of sulfur-containing by-products. These have medicinal properties, but most are not antibiotic.

The easiest method is to take garlic cloves orally, although some reports indicate that pain can also be relieved by locally rubbing the area with cloves of garlic. Garlic oil is rapidly absorbed through the skin and into the blood stream to reach the affected areas.

Heart Attacks

Professor Hams Reuter of Cologne University says that there is proof that garlic helps break up cholesterol in blood vessels, thus preventing hardening of arteries which can lead to heart attack. Taking garlic after a heart attack also brings down the cholesterol levels however the earlier damage may not be repaired but garlic consumption will minimise the chances of new attacks.[1]

Cancer

Garlic preparations, including extracts and juices, have been used successfully against cancer in both animal and human studies, says Dr. Paavo Airola, a naturopathic physician and nutritionist. In one controlled study of mice infected with cancer cells, some were treated with garlic extract and some were not. The mice not given garlic died within 16 days while the others lived for six months. Recent studies done in Russia have found garlic preparations to retard tumour in human beings, writes Dr. Airola.[2]

Skin Disorders

Garlic has also been used successfully for a variety of skin disorders. Pimples disappear without scar when rubbed with raw garlic several

> According to a report in the *Journal of Agriculture and Food Chemistry* (2003), garlic skin contains powerful antioxidant properties; there are six antioxidant compounds within its skin. Peeling garlic removes phenylpropanoid antioxidants in its velvety membrane which help fight the ageing process and protects the heart.

1. M.K Kaul Mirror, *Monthly Magazine*, Bombay, pp. 40, June 1986 issue.
2. Ibid.

times a day. The external use of garlic helps to clear the skin of spots, pimples and boils. The process is helped by taking garlic orally to purify the blood-stream for long-term clearer skin. A regular course of two garlic cloves a day helps clear minor skin infections quickly.

Wounds and Ulcers

Garlic juice with three parts of distilled water has been used to cleanse infected wounds. Definite improvement is noticed within 24 hours and substantial improvement within 48 hours.[1] Application of dressing containing 15 per cent garlic juice once a day over an ulcer removes pus within a few days. It also relieves pain.

Diphtheria

Garlic is an excellent remedy for diphtheria. Chewing about 30 to 60 gms of garlic regularly removes the membranes, reduces temperature and brings relief to the patient. After the membranes disappear, the same quantity of garlic should be chewed once daily. The diphtheria patient has no taste or smell and merely finds the garlic hot.[2]

Whooping Cough

Syrup of garlic is recommended in doses of five drops to a teaspoonful two or three times a day for whooping cough. It should be given more often if the coughing spells are frequent and violent.[3]

Sexual Debility

Garlic is a natural aphrodisiac. Dr. Robinson, an eminent sexologist of America considers it so. It is a tonic for restoring loss of sexual power, sexual debility, impotency from over indulgence in sex and nervous exhaustion. It is said to be especially useful to old men of high nervous tension and diminishing sexual power.[4]

---

1. Col. R.N. Chopra, *Indigenous Drugs of India*, pp. 273, Acadeinio Publishers, Calcutta, 1982.
2. Ibid.
3. Dr. S.J. Singh, *Food Remedies*, pp. 91, Nature Cure Council of Medical Research. Lucknow, 1982.
4. Ibid, pp. 92

Uses

Garlic like onions, leeks, and various other garden flowers belongs to the plant of genus called Allium. It is the most widely used of the cultivated alliums after onions. It is used both as a food and as a seasoning in soups, sauces and pickles.

Garlic, Raw or Cooked. Which is better?

Fresh raw garlic is undoubtedly the best!

Heating garlic dramatically reduces its antibiotic effect. While many medicinal effects remain in heated garlic tea or cooked garlic in food, its antibiotic properties are lost. The antibiotic properties of garlic oil are completely destroyed after heating for twenty minutes. Garlic slowly loses its antibiotic properties in storage.

Some ways of taking garlic orally are:

- Chew a clove of raw, chopped or crushed garlic. Oral raw garlic kills infectious bacteria in the intestines directly.
- Blend a clove in a cup of water or milk and drink it.
- Blend it in one-half cup of carrot juice.
- Put the chopped or crushed clove in a cup of already cooked soup or rice.
- Squeeze juice of one lemon; peel and cut in half three to five cloves of garlic, and combine this and lemon juice in one cup of water, add a little powdered or fresh ginger and some honey, and blend to a smooth mixture. Drink the whole thing at one go.

Cooked Garlic: slice a whole garlic head in half lengthwise or even roast whole. Drizzle with olive oil, then add to your baking tray when baking vegetables.

GINGER

Botanical Name: *Zingiber officinalse*
Indian Name: *Adrak*

Ginger is a perennial herb, with underground branching stems called rhizomes which are white or yellow and become grey-brown or orange with age, and are upto 2.5 cm in diameter. Leaves and rhizomes have a characteristic fragrant odour when cut or bruised. Rhizomes are dug out after the leafy parts are dry. They are sold as fresh ginger or are peeled and dried. The sun-dried ginger is commonly known as *sounth* in India.

Origin and Distribution: Ginger is believed to have originated in India and appears to have been used as a spice and a medicine from the early times. There are numerous references to ginger in Sanskrit literature and in Chinese medical treatises. It was known in Europe in the first century and mentioned by Dioscorides and Pliny and soon spread to all tropical countries. The sanskrit name *singebera* gave rise to the Greek *Zingiberi* and to later to *Zingiber* in Latin.

Natural Benefits and Curative Properties

Ginger has been used as medicine in India from the Vedic period and is called *maha-aushadhi*, meaning a great medicine. Ancient physicians used ginger as a carminative and as an anti-fermenting medicine. Galen, the Greek physician, used ginger to rectify defective humours of the body including in the treatment of paralysis caused by phlegmatic imbalance in the body. Avicenna, another physician used it as an aphrodisiac.

Ginger*

Food Value		**Minerals and Vitamins**	
Moisture	80.9%	Calcium	20 mg
Protein	2.3%	Phosphorus	60 mg
Fat	0.9%	Iron	2.6 mg
Minerals	1.2%	Vitamin C	6 mg
Fibre	2.4%	Small amounts of	
Carbohydrates	12.3%	Vitamin B Complex	
	100%		

**Values per 100 gms edible portion | Calorific Value - 67*

Even today ginger is widely used in traditional medicine in India and the far East. Taken internally, it is a stimulating carminative and applied locally it acts as a rubefacient and counter-irritant. Like many other spices, ginger is believed to have aphrodisiac properties.

Ginger yields an essential oil, but since it lacks the pungent principle, it is used in manufacturing of flavouring essence and perfumery. An oleoresin i.e. a mixture of oil and resin is also extracted from ginger in which full pungency of the spice is preserved; it is used both for flavouring and for medicinal purposes.

Digestive System Disorders

Ginger is a valuable drug for treating dyspepsia, flatulence, colic, vomiting, spasms nausea, including post surgery nausea and nausea in cancer patients and other painful affections of the stomach and the bowels. Chewing a piece of fresh ginger after meals regularly is an insurance against these ailments. This protective action is attributable to excessive secretion of saliva, diastase enzyme and volatile oil.

Half a teaspoon of fresh ginger juice, mixed with one teaspoonful each of fresh lime juice and fresh mint juice and a tablespoonful of honey, constitutes an effective medicine for dyspepsia, nausea and vomiting resulting from biliousness, indigestion, morning sickness,

Superfood in Every Kitchen

Ginger is often called a "superfood" — and for good reason!

Ginger contains a very high nutritional density per portion. Besides being a delicious spice for cooking, ginger has powerful health benefits, such as anti-inflammatory, antibacterial and antiviral properties. It contains *gingerol* as its main bioactive component, which is responsible for most of its medicinal properties. Dried ginger, which is scraped or peeled before drying, constitutes the spice, and is valued for its flavour, pungency, aroma and medicinal value. It is widely used in Indian cooking.

hepatitis or jaundice and piles. This mixture should be sucked thrice daily in treatment of these conditions.[1]

Cough and Cold

Ginger's warming effect and healing properties make it an excellent remedy for coughs and colds. Juice of ginger with honey is advised three or four times a day in case of cough. In case of colds, ginger should be cut into small pieces and boiled in a cup of water, strained, half a teaspoon of sugar added and taken while hot. Ginger tea, prepared by adding few pieces of crushed ginger into boiled water before adding tea leaves, is also an effective remedy.

Respiratory Disorders

A teaspoonful of the fresh ginger juice mixed with a cupful of fenugreek decoction and honey is an excellent diaphoretic mixture which increases sweating to reduce fever in influenza. It acts as an expectorant in bronchitis, asthma, whooping cough and tuberculosis of the lungs.[2]

Aches and Pains

Ginger is an excellent pain killer. It can cure all types of pain. An ointment made by rubbing dry ginger with a little water and applied to forehead relieves headache. It allays tooth ache when applied to the face. In case of earache, a few drops of ginger juice give relief.

Sexual Debility

Ginger juice is a valuable aphrodisiac. Half a teaspoon of ginger juice taken with a half-boiled egg and honey, once daily at night for a month tones up the sex centres and cures impotency, premature ejaculation, spermatorrhea.

Menstrual Disorders

A piece of fresh ginger pounded and boiled in a cupful of water for few minutes, sweetened with sugar should be taken thrice daily after meals as a medicine for dysmenorrhoea and amenorrhoea due to exposure to cold winds and taking cold bath.[3]

---

1. Ibid., pp. 607.
2. Ibid., pp. 608.
3. Hakeem Mahamood Shariff, *Zathi Tajrubath*, Urdu MS Chamraj Nagar, 1968.

Uses

Ginger is a widely-used spice making gingerbread, biscuits, cakes, puddings, soups and pickles, as curry powder and to prepare ginger beer, ginger ale and ginger wine. It was earlier much used for spicing wines, possets and porter, the last one often being stirred with a red-hot poker.

LETTUCE

Botanical Name: *Lactuca sativa*
Indian Names: *Kahu or Kasmi-sāg, Salād pattā*

Lettuce is known as the king of salad plants. It has rounded leaves upto 25 cms in length and 15 cms in width. There are several varieties of lettuce, differing in colour of the leaves, size and texture. The colour of leaves varies from light to dark green. Generally only two varieties are used in salads, namely, the loose-leaf lettuce and the true head-lettuce. In the loose-leaf lettuce the leaves hang on all sides. The head-lettuce is like a cabbage with its leaves drawn together.

Origin and Distribution: The original home of lettuce appears to be the Middle-East. The first records of lettuce in a long-leaved form are depicted on Egyptian tombs dated 4500 BC. It was used by the Persian royalty more than 550 BC.

Lettuce reached China in the seventh century AD and England in 1520. King Henry VIII is said to have conferred a special reward upon the gardener who devised the combination of lettuce and cherries for the royal table. Lettuce is comparatively a recent introduction into the tropics. It is now widely cultivated in India, Malaysia, Indonesia, the Philippines, China, the Caribbean, Central and South America and Africa.

Food Value: Lettuce is rich in vitamin content, especially the antiscorbutic vitamin C. It is bulky, low in food value but ranks high for its health properties. It is rich in mineral salts with alkaline

Lettuce*

Food Value		Minerals and Vitamins	
Moisture	93.4%	Calcium	50 mg
Protein	2.1%	Phosphorus	28 mg
Fat	0.3%	Iron	2.4 mg
Minerals	1.2%	Vitamin C	10 mg
Fibre	0.5%	Small amounts of	
Carbohydrates	2.5%	Vitamin B Complex	
	100%		

**Values per 100 gms edible portion | Calorific Value - 42*

elements predominating. This helps to keep the blood clean, the mind alert and the body in good health.

The loose-leaf lettuce is considered a better food than the head-lettuce. It has the advantage of being more exposed to sunlight, thus providing it with a richer supply of vitamins than the head-lettuce in which the leaves are closed. Irrespective of the variety selected, it should be fresh, crisp and green-leafed. The greener the leaves, the higher is the vitamin content.

Natural Benefits and Curative Properties

Lettuce contains several health-building and medicinal properties. It is good for the brain, the nervous system and the lungs. The raw juice of lettuce is cool and refreshing. The high content of magnesium in the juice revitalises the muscle tissues, the nerves and the brain.

While preparing lettuce juice, especially for therapeutic purposes, leaves of the darker shade of green should be preferred. The leaves which are inside the head of lettuce are on the lighter side and should be discarded. The former are much richer in chlorophyll and other vital elements than the latter.

Constipation

Being rich in cellulose, lettuce increases the bulk of intestinal contents and encourages peristalsis. It is, therefore, highly beneficial in curing chronic constipation.

Insomnia

Lettuce is beneficial in treating insomnia; it contains a sleep inducing substance called "lectucarium". According to Culpepper, the ancient English herbalist, juice of lettuce mixed with oil of roses, applied to the forehead and temples, induces sleep and eases headaches.[1] A decoction of lettuce seeds is useful in insomnia and wakefulness resulting from mental overwork.

Diabetes

Lettuce is amongst the important foods prescribed for the diabetics. It belongs to that select group of vegetables which contain three per cent or less of carbohydrates.

Anaemia

Lettuce contains considerable amount of iron and a good form of vegetable haemoglobin. It is therefore a good tonic food for anaemia. The iron obtained is absorbed by the body to a much greater degree than the inorganic iron tonic.

Pregnancy and Lactation

Eating raw lettuce is highly beneficial during pregnancy and lactation. An important nutritional factor, folic acid, in lettuce prevents megaloblastic anaemia during pregnancy. In a series of experiments it was confirmed that pregnant mothers who had lettuce regularly were free from nutritional anaemia. Lettuce is believed to have a great influence over the secretion of progesterone hormone. Eating lettuce with spinach, peas, asparagus and cauliflower increases the folic acid or vitamin B content of the food. It is estimated that about 300-500 mcg. of this vitamin is required daily in the last trimester;[2] deficiency can cause megaloblastic anaemia.

Uses

Lettuce is normally used raw as salad. Loose-leaf lettuce is also cooked as a green vegetable. It cooks without adding water; the water which clings after washing suffices. It should be kept covered over a stove for the first few minutes until the juice starts flowing and then cooked uncovered for about 10 minutes.

---

1. Susane E. Charmaine, *The Complete Raw Juice Therapy*, pp. 78 Thorsons Publishing Group, Great Britain, 1987.
2. Dr. Aman, *Medicinal Secrets of Your Food*, pp. 360, Indo-American Hospital, Mysore, 1985.

Precautions: Lettuce leaves should be washed thoroughly leaf by leaf before use. After washing these leaves should be put within the folds of a clean towel until the leaves are completely dry.

MINT

Botanical Name: *Minthe spicata*
Indian Name: *Pudina*

Mint is a popular spice used extensively in India. It is an erect, branched perennial herb with modified underground stems. The shoots produced from these stems are four-angled, and bear oval-shaped leaves which are simple, delicate, thin, dark green in colour and fragrant.

Origin and Distribution: Mint is a native of temperate Europe. Ancient Romans and Greeks knew about this plant. The story goes that Minthe, the damsel lover of God Pluto, was transferred into this herb by Persephone's anger, the Goddess of Wealth and Pluto's wife. Therefore mint is commonly known as Minthae in Latin. The ancient Greek physician, Saufarsats, used mint in preparing various carminative medicines. Even Islamic physicians were familiar with this herb. Chinese and Japanese knew of this herb almost two thousand years go.[1]

Food Value: Mint contains plenty of vitamins and is rich in several minerals. The fresh and dried leaves are used for mint sauce and jelly and to flavour foods. Mint oil is used in flavouring chewing gum, tooth paste and in confectionery and pharmaceutical preparations.

Natural Benefits and Curative Properties

Mint is much valued as a carminative for relieving gastric discomfort, as a stimulant, as an antispasmodic to relieve muscle strain and

1. Dr. Aman, *Medicinal Secrets of Your Food*, pp. 363, Indo American Hospital, Mysore, 1985.

Mint*

Food Value		Minerals and Vitamins	
Moisture	84.9%	Calcium	200 mg
Protein	4.8%	Phosphorus	62 mg
Fat	0.6%	Iron	15.6 mg
Minerals	1.9%	Vitamin C	27 mg
Fibre	2.0%	Small amounts of Vit B Complex and good amount of Vit D and E	
Carbohydrates	5.8%		
	100%		

**Values per 100 gms edible portion | Calorific Value - 48*

as a stomachic for improving appetite. The digestive properties of mint make it an ingredient of most drugs prescribed for stomach ailments. It is good for the liver and helps dissolve gravel in kidneys and bladder.

Digestive Disorders

Mint juice is a good appetiser. Fresh mint leaf juice mixed with a teaspoonful of lime juice and honey is given thrice a day for treating indigestion, biliousness, flatulent colic, thread worms, morning sickness and summer diarrhoea.

According to the well-known Naturopath father Kneipp, 'A cupful of mint tea taken every morning and evening assists digestion and gives a fresh and healthy appearance. Mint powder renders the same service, if one or two pinches are taken daily in the food or in water.' He also claims that milk or tea prepared with mint and taken warm, relieves abdominal pains.[1]

The seeds of mint are beneficial in relieving severe abdominal pain due to indigestion in growing children. The child can be given a quarter teaspoonful of the seeds to chew and swallow with water in such conditions.

Respiratory Disorders

A teaspoonful of fresh mint juice, mixed with two spoonfuls of pure malt vinegar and equal quantity of honey stirred in about 150 ml of carrot juice and given thrice daily acts as a medicinal tonic during

1. Dr. S.J. Singh, *Food Remedies*, pp. 142, Nature Cure Council of Medical Research, Lucknow, 1982.

treatment of tuberculosis, asthma and bronchitis. It liquifies the sputum, nourishes the lungs, increases resistance against infection and counteracts adverse effects of anti-tubercular drugs. It prevents asthmatic attacks and reduces congestion in air passages.

Oral Disorders

Fresh leaves of mint chewed daily are an effective antiseptic dentifrice i.e. tooth paste. The chlorophyll combined with other antiseptic chemicals in the mint kills foul-odour causing germs and strengthens gums by providing nutrients thus preventing tooth decay, pyorrhoea, pre-mature fall of the teeth etc. It also keeps the mouth fresh and improves the sense of taste.

Hoarseness

Gargling with a decoction of fresh with salt cures hoarseness resulting from shouting or singing loudly. If used prior to singing it keeps the voice clear and is therefore a boon to singers and orators.[1]

> You are what you eat;
> eating junk food isn't a reward.
> It is a punishment.

Skin Disorders

Application of fresh mint juice over face every night cures pimples and prevents dry skin. Juice applied on insect stings, eczema, scabies and contact dermatitis speeds up healing.

Natural Birth-Control

In *Ayurveda*, powdered dry mint is regarded as a harmless herb for birth control. It is believed that a woman swallowing 10 gms of mint powder before sexual intercourse will not conceive long as she continues this practice. The mint should be dried in shade, powdered and bottled.[2]

---

1. Ibid, pp. 369.
2. Kvj. Ganpati Singh Verma, *Miracles of Indian Herbism*, p. 115, Rasayan Pharmacy, New Delhi, 1982.

ONION

Botanical Name: *Allium cepa*
Indian Name: *Piyāz*

Onion, a pungent edible of the lily family, is one of the earliest cultivated vegetables and considered a food of exceptional value. It is also widely used for flavouring and seasoning.

Onion is a biennial herb, usually grown as an annual. When crushed it produces a strong odour. It has a superficial root system, a very short and flattened stem at the base of the plant which increases in diameter as it grows. When the plant reaches a certain stage of growth a bulb is formed by thickening of the leaf bases. The fruit is a globular capsule.

Origin and Cultivation: Onion is believed to have originated in Central Asia. It has been cultivated as a food since the ancient times in the Middle East and India. In Egypt, it has been found depicted on tombs dating as early as 3200 BC.

The Sanskrit for onion is *palandu* which is mentioned in the *Garuda Purana*. The great Indian sages, Maharishi Atreya and Lord Dhanwantri, have described the use of onions in detail. It is referred to in the Bible; the Israelites remembered onions they ate in Egypt when being led by Moses to the land of Canaan in about 1500 BC.

It is on record that the Jews loved onions so much that they named a city after it — Onion. This city was built in 173 BC near the Gulf of Suez. The man who built it was called Onions. The city existed for 343 years.

Onion is cultivated in most parts of the world, including India, Myanmar, Malaysia, Indonesia, Philippines, China, Egypt, West and East Africa, tropical America and the Caribbean.

Food Value: Onion, which derives its name from the Latin *Onio* and French *Oignon*, has been described as a dynamite amongst natural foods. Compared with other fresh vegetables, it is relatively high in food value, moderate in protein content and rich in calcium and riboflavin. There is considerable variation in composition between its varieties, which changes with the stage of maturity and the length of storage.

The odour of onion is due to organic sulphur compounds, which is produced only when the tissues are cut or injured[1]. Heating, freezing and drying prevents the enzyme action. That is why cooking produces a different odour, flavour and pungency. The pungent flavour of onion is much appreciated in many countries. A strong odour lingers for a considerable time after eating onions; it is said that the small particles retained in the mouth which cannot always be removed by brushing give this odour.

Onion*

Food Value		**Minerals and Vitamins**	
Moisture	86.6%	Calcium	47 mg
Protein	1.2%	Phosphorus	50 mg
Fat	0.1%	Iron	0.7 mg
Minerals	0.6%	Vitamin C	11 mg
Fibre	0.4%	Small amounts of	
Carbohydrates	11.1%	Vitamin B Complex	
	100%		

**Values per 100 gms edible portion | Calorific Value - 51*

Onion has a good keeping quality. Dried cured bulbs can be kept for several months without deterioration and can stand rough handling. Long storage life is usually associated with high pungency.

Natural Benefits and Curative Properties

Onion is highly valued for its therapeutic properties. It has been used as a food remedy since times immemorial. The physicians of ancient Egypt prescribed onions in various diseases. Dioscorides in the first century AD attributed many remedies to the plant — as a stimulant, a diuretic, an expectorant and a rubefacient.

White onion is preferable to the red and yellow varieties. Onions should be taken with meals preferably raw; fried or cooked onions are comparatively difficult to digest. For therapeutic purposes, it is advisable to use onion juice for its all round medicinal properties.

1. Produced by enzyme action on a water-soluble amino acid.

Being a stimulating and irritating food, excess consumption of onions should be avoided.

Several parts of the plant have a place in the traditional medicine. The seeds of onion increase semen and provide relief from dental worms and urinary diseases. The stalks of onion are a source of Vitamin A, thiamin and ascorbic acid. They are used both when tender and mature.

Respiratory Disease

Onion is said to possess expectorant properties. It liquifies phlegm and prevents any further formation. For centuries it has been used as a food remedy in colds, cough, bronchitis and influenza. Three to four teaspoons of equal amounts of onion juice and honey mixed together are advised daily. It is one of the safest preventive medicines against common cold during winter.

Tooth Disorders

Latest researches of Russian doctors have confirmed the bactericidal properties of onion. These researches conclude that one raw onion consumed daily after thorough mastication, protects against a host of teeth disorders. Dr. B.P. Tohkin of Russia, who contributed to this research, says that chewing raw onion for three minutes is sufficient to kill all germs present in the mouth. Toothache is often allayed by placing a small piece of onion on the bad tooth or gum.

Anaemia

Onions are noted for their easily assimilable iron content. They are, therefore, beneficial in treating anaemia.

Heart Disease

Dr. N.N. Gupta of the K.G. Medical College, Lucknow, in 1966, and a 1968 panel of doctors in England have stated that onion is beneficial in diseases of the heart; these benefits are due to the presence of an essential oil, aliypropyl disulphide, catechol, protocatechnic acid, thiopropiono aldehyde, thiocyanate, calcium, iron, phosphorus and vitamins in onion.

A long research by Dr. N. Radhakrishnan of Trivandrum Medical College and Dr. K. Madhavan Kutty has established that onions were very valuable remedy in heart diseases; they correct thrombosis and reduce blood cholesterol.[1]

Sexual Debility

As an aphrodisiac, onion is second only to garlic. It increases libido and strengthens reproductory organs. White variety of onion, peeled, crushed and fried in pure butter, taken regularly with a spoonful of honey on empty stomach acts as an excellent aphrodisiac. The powder of black gram when dipped in juice of onion for seven days and dried, produces a mixture called *kanji*. This also acts an aphrodisiac.[2]

Skin Disorders

Onion irritates the skin circulation and stimulates blood circulation in the mucous membrane. Sometimes even warts can disappear if rubbed with cut onions. Roasted or otherwise, onions are applied as a poultice to boils, bruises, wounds, etc., to bring boils to maturity.

Ear Disorders

Warm onion juice dipped on cotton wool and put into the ear is a popular Russian remedy for ringing in the ears. It can also relieves earache.

Cholera

Onion is an effective remedy for cholera. About 30 gms of onion and seven black peppers finely pounded in a pestle is advised for a patient of cholera. It allays thirst and restlessness and the patient feels better. It also immediately lessens vomiting and diarrhoea. Adding a little sugar increases its efficacy.[3]

Urinary System Disorders

Onions are highly beneficial in treating urinary system disorders. For burning sensation in urine, six grams of onion should be boiled in 500 ml of water till half the water evaporates, strained, allowed

---

1. Dr. S.J. Singh, *Food Remedies*, pp. 1 16 Nature Cure Council of Medical Research, Lucknow, 1982.
2. 'Treatment by Onions for Cure and Prevention of Disease', Prakritrani, Monthly Magazine, January, 1988. pp. 9.
3. Ibid., p. 10.

to cool and given to the patient. This relieves burning sensation in urine. Onion rubbed in water and mixed with 60 gms of sugar is helpful in retention of urine. It brings about free urination within a short time.[1]

Piles, Bleeding

Onions are valuable in healing bleeding piles. About 30 gms of onions should be finely rubbed in water and 60 gms of sugar added to it. Taken twice daily brings relief within a few days.

Uses

Immature and mature bulbs of onions are eaten raw or may be cooked and eaten as a vegetable. They can used in soups and sauces and as seasoning in food. Coated with gram flour and fried, onion *bhajiya* makes an excellent snack. Small white leaf at the base of the plant (where the bulb starts) are eaten raw in salads. These immature plants are known as green or spring onions. Onion oil, produced by steam distillation, is used to a limited extent for flavouring foods.

In recent years, there has been an increasing demand for dehydrated onion products. Sliced and dried onions are used for flavouring food and in canned meat products, sausages, canned and dried soups and ketchups. Dried onion flakes can be reconstituted by cooking in water and used. Chopped and dried green onion tops may be used as a substitute for chives — a commonly used herb which is used as a flavouring herb.

POTATO

Botanical Name: *Solanum tuberosum*
Indian Name: *Alu*

Potato is an annual plant with swollen underground stem tubers. It perhaps the most widely used vegetable in the world, an indispensable item of daily food and nutrition.

1. Kvj. Ganpati Singh Verma, *Miracles of Onions*, pp. 16. Rasayan Pharmacy, Delhi, 1981.

Origin and Distribution: Potato is a native of South America. It was introduced in Europe in the later-half of the 16th century, where for nearly one hundred years it was looked upon as a poisonous tuber. Its food value was realised only in 1771, when a prize was offered in France for discovering food which could be used as substitute for wheat in times of famine.

In the United States, potato was introduced by the Irish immigrants in 1719. The Spaniards took it to Philippines at an early date. It came to India in the 17th century. In volume, potato exceeds all other crops grown in the world.

Food Value: Potato has high nutritive value. Its chief food principle is starch, but it has a notable amount of protein of high biological value. It is rich in soda, potash, vitamins A and B and a substantial amount of alkaline salts.

Potato*

Food Value		**Minerals and Vitamins**	
Moisture	74.7%	Calcium	10 mg
Protein	1.6%	Phosphorus	40 mg
Fat	0.1%	Iron	0.7 mg
Minerals	0.6%	Vitamin C	17 mg
Fibre	0.4%	Small amounts of	
Carbohydrates	22.6%	Vitamin B Complex	
	100%		

**Values per 100 gms edible portion | Calorific Value - 97*

Potato can be boiled, baked, steamed and cooked with other vegetables. However potatoes should always be cooked with skin; the most nutritive part of a potato lies just below its skin and it is rich in protein and mineral salts.

Natural Benefits and Curative Properties

Potato contains several medicinal virtues. It is one of the most strongly alkaline of all foods, and therefore, very helpful in maintaining the alkali reserve of the body. This makes it a natural antidote for overdose of acid or acidosis. It dissolves uric acid and lime. It also prevents fermentation in intestines and promotes growth of friendly bacteria in the digestive tract.

Potatoes should be avoided by the obese; they are fattening. They should also be excluded from the diet of those suffering from venereal diseases or with aphrodisiac tendencies. The vegetable contains an alkaloid toxin known as solanine which affects the nerves controlling the sexual organs. The solanine poison is particularly presents in potatoes which are green. The combination of cooked meat and potatoes intensifies the solanine poison, which together with presence of uric acid crystals resulting from ingestion of meat may cause excessive irritation of sexual organs.

Potato Therapy

An exclusive diet of potatoes is considered valuable in treating chronic constipation, intestinal toxaemia, uric acid diseases, renal calculi or stone, and dropsy. If needed this diet can be employed with beneficial results for several months. Potatoes can be consumed baked, steamed and in soups. Other vegetables which can be taken when on this diet are spinach, beet tops, turnip tops, cucumber, lettuce, celery, tomatoes and other green vegetables.

Scurvy

Potato is an excellent food remedy in scurvy. It has been noted in history of medicine that scurvy in Europe became more and more uncommon with the progress of potato cultivation and made its appearance only when the crop failed. Dr. G.F. Still used "potato

Potato Skin is Nutrition Rich

You double your intake of nutrients by eating potato skin. Just one fist-sized potato skin provides half your RDA (Recommended Daily Allowance) of soluble fire, potassium, phosphorous, iron, zinc and vitamin C. Potatoes contain more vitamin C than oranges, so are perfect for anyone warding off colds and boosting immunity.

How to eat it: Roast unpeeled potato wedges in a drizzle of olive oil.

cream" in curing cases of infantile scurvy, while Dr. A.F. Hess used ordinary mashed potatoes for the same purposes.[1]

Rheumatism

One or two teaspoonful of the juice pressed from mashed raw potatoes taken before meals is an excellent remedy for rheumatism. This helps eliminate acid in the body and relieve rheumatism. In some rural areas of Great Britain, it was a custom for rheumatic sufferer to carry a potato in their pocket in the belief that the potato would absorb some of the acid from the sufferer's body.

The skin of the potato is also an excellent food remedy for rheumatism. It is exceptionally rich in vital mineral salts, and even the water in which the peelings have been boiled is an effective remedy for ailments caused by excess acid in the system. Potato peelings should be thoroughly washed and boiled for few minutes, the decoction strained and a glassful taken three or four times daily.[2]

Digestive System Disorders

Stomach ulcers can be successfully treated with juice of raw pink potatoes. Potato juice also relieves gastritis. The recommended dose is half a cupful half an hour before meals. Potato starch is administered as an anti-inflammatory for gastro-intestinal diseases and toxins.

Skin Blemishes

Juice of raw potatoes helps clear skin blemishes. The high content of potassium, sulphur, phosphorus and chlorine in the potato helps cleanse these blemishes. These elements are, however, of value only in raw potatoes; raw potatoes are composed of live organic atoms. Cooked, these get converted into inorganic atoms and are of little value for constructive purposes.[3]

The juicy pulp of shredded raw potatoes can be applied as a poultice in clearing wrinkles and other skin blemishes caused by the

---

1. Dr. S.J. Singh, *Food Remedies*, pp. 174, Nature Cure Council of Medical Research, Lucknow, 1982.
2. Eric F.W. Powell, *Health from the Kitchen*, pp. 20, Health Science Press, England, 1973.
3. N.W. Walker, *Raw Vegetable Juices*. pp. 77, Jove Books. New York, 1983.

ageing process. It may be rubbed on the face and other portions of body that have wrinkles before retiring at night. This helps 'melt' the wrinkles, banish age spots and clear the skin. The enzymes in raw potato pulp, combined with the Vitamin C and the natural starch, help create a 'skin food' that nourishes the starved cellular tissues of the skin. Also the alkaline juice of the potato promote an antiseptic action that gives a glowing look. Much of the decaying skin sloughs off by the acid portion of the pulp.[1]

Swellings

Applied externally, raw potato juice is valuable in treating swellings and other disorders of joints and muscles. After extraction, the juice should be boiled down to about one-fifth its original quantity, and a little glycerine added as a preservative. This is used as a liniment. It should be applied after fomentation of the affected parts and repeated every three hours until pain and swelling are relieved.

RADISH

Botanical Name: *Raphanus sativus*
Indian Name: *Mooli*

Radish is one of the most commonly used vegetables in India. It is a hairy annual herb with only one root which is round, cylindrical or tapering, white or red, slightly coarse, fleshy, succulent, and 3 to 7 cm thick, 10 to 20 cm long with a pungent flavour. It stimulates appetite and promotes a healthy bloodstream.

There are many varieties of radish, differing in size and colour. The red and white coloured are the most familiar. They are tender when young but become woody and tough as they mature.

Origin and Distribution: Radish is believed to have originated in West Asia and was cultivated in ancient Egypt, Greece and Rome.

1. Carlson Wade, *Health Secrets from the Orient*, pp. 65, Allied Publishers, Delhi.

Its areas of cultivation include South America, East and West Africa, the Caribbean, Malaysia, India, and most tropical areas.

Food Value: Radish is one of the richest sources of iron, calcium and sodium amongst the common vegetables. The roots, rather than the leaves of small plants, are generally used as a food item. For maximum benefit they should be eaten raw. Cooking destroys the vitamin content and its powerful antiscorbutic properties. Radish leaves have more calcium, phosphorus, vitamin C and protein than the radish itself. The leaves are also eaten as salad or used in cooking.

Radish*

Food Value		**Minerals and Vitamins**	
Moisture	94.4%	Calcium	35 mg
Protein	0.7%	Phosphorus	22 mg
Fat	0.1%	Iron	0.4 mg
Minerals	0.6%	Vitamin C	15 mg
Fibre	0.8%	Small amounts of	
Carbohydrates	3.4%	Vitamin B Complex	
	100%		

Calorific Value - 17

Radish Leaves*

Food Value		**Minerals and Vitamins**	
Moisture	90.8%	Calcium	265 mg
Protein	3.8%	Phosphorus	59 mg
Fat	0.4%	Iron	3.6 mg
Minerals	1.6%	Vitamin C	81 mg
Fibre	1.0%	Small amounts of	
Carbohydrates	2.4%	Vitamin B Complex	
	100%		

**Values per 100 gms edible portion | Calorific Value - 28*

Natural Benefits and Curative Properties

Radish leaves are diuretic, antiscorbutic and laxative. The tap root is strongly antiscorbutic and prevents and cures scurvy. The seeds are expectorant, diuretic, laxative and a stimulant and being carminative relieve gastric discomforts.

Piles

The juice and the fresh root are regarded as an effective remedy. It should be given in doses of 60 to 90 ml morning and evening.

Genito-Urinary Disorders

Juice is also beneficial in treating dysuria or painful urination, and strangury or severe urethral pain. It can be given in doses mentioned above and repeated as often as necessary. A cupful of radish leaf-juice given once daily for a fortnight acts as a curative medicine in dissolving any gravel in urinary tract and for treating cystitis i.e. inflammation of urinary bladder.

Chest Complaints

A syrup prepared by mixing a teaspoonful of fresh radish juice with equal quantity of honey and a little rock salt is highly beneficial in the treatment of hoarse throat, whooping cough, bronchial disorders and other chest complaints. It should be given thrice daily.

Hepatitis/Jaundice

Green leaves of radish are beneficial in treating jaundice. The leaves are pounded, their juice expressed and finely sieved. It should be sweetened to taste by adding fine crystalline sugar. About half a kg of this juice should be taken daily by an adult patient for immediate relief. The preparation induces healthy appetite and proper evacuation of bowels which gradually reduces the problem.[1]

Leucoderma

A paste made from the seeds of radish is valuable in leucoderma. About 35 gm of seeds are powdered in vinegar and applied on the white patches of leucoderma. For better results seeds should be finely pounded along with a pinch of arsenic poison and soaked in vinegar at night. This paste should be rubbed on the white patches of leucoderma.[2] This preparation is for external use only.

Other Skin Disorders

Radish seeds contain a bleaching substance and an emulsion made of seeds with water applied on the face removes black heads and freckles. It can be applied with benefit in treating ringworm.[3]

---

1. Kvj. Ganpati Singh Verma, *Miracles of Indian Herbs*, pp. 56 Rasayan Pharmacy, New Delhi; 1982.
2. Ibid., p. 92
3. Dr. Aman, *Medicinal Secrets of Your Foods*, pp. 163. Indo American Hospital, Mysore, 1985.

SOYABEAN

Botanical Name: *Glycine max*
Indian Name: *Bhat, Soyabean*

Soyabean is one of the most nutritious foods. It belongs to the family of legumes or pulses and is perhaps one of the earliest amongst the cultivated crops.

Soyabean is one of the most important sources of oil and protein. It is an annual plant which grows upto 150 cms in height with alternate leaves and grey, brown or black, pods, borne in clusters. Seeds are more or less round, and yellow, green, brown or black in colour.

Origin and Distribution: The name soya has its origin in the Chinese word *shu* and *sou*. The Aryans of Central Asia offered soya along with honey as a sacred food to the departed. The yogis of Indus Valley Civilisation supplemented their meatless diet with this soyabean to make up for any deficiency of good protein.

Soyabean is a native of the Far East. It has been referred to in a Chinese book written by Emperor Shen Nung of China as early as 2838 BC. The plant was given so much importance that even the Emperor would sow it with great pomp every year. It is now a popular crop and widely cultivated in the United States, Europe, South Africa, Russia, Australia and other countries. In the recent years several countries like Brazil, Rumania and Argentina have substantially increased their soyabean production. India too has joined the 'soyabean race' and there is growing awareness of the potential benefits and uses of soyabean.

Food Value: Soyabean is esteemed for its high food value. It is a valuable source of protein, vitamins, minerals and other food ingredients. It contains vitamin B complex, biotin, folic acid, pantothenic acid, pyridoxine and vitamin E.

Soyabean is particularly valued for its 'complete' protein content. It contains all essential amino acids or building blocks of protein in

Soyabean*

Food Value		Minerals and Vitamins	
Moisture	8.1%	Calcium	240 mg
Protein	43.2%	Phosphorus	690 mg
Fat	19.5%	Iron	11.5 mg
Minerals	3.7%	Small amounts of	
Fibre	4.6%	Vitamin B Complex	
Carbohydrates	20.9%	and Vitamin E	
	100%		

**Values per 100 gms edible portion | Calorific Value - 432*

the proportions that make it most valuable for human needs. It is the best of all vegetable proteins and has more protein than milk, eggs and meat.

Natural Benefit and Curative Properties

Soyabean contains many medicinal virtues. While most proteins are acid in their ash, soyabean is rich in alkaline bearing salts and hence regarded as a corrective diet. The Chinese who consume soyabeans liberally believe that it makes the body plump, improves complexion, stimulates growth, prevents constipation and many other physical ailments. Research in Europe and America has corroborated much of these claims.

Soyabean, especially in the form of milk, is highly beneficial. This milk is prepared by soaking the beans in water for about 12 hours. The skin of the beans is then removed and the beans ground into a fine paste, mixed with water, three times its quantity. The mixture is then boiled on slow fire, stirring it frequently. After cooling, it is strained through a fine sieve and sugar added to it.

For children, soyabean milk is at par with cow's milk in nutrient content. Investigations have shown that 90 per cent of the soyabean protein is absorbed in the body and 95 to 100 per cent of the milk is digested. It is very helpful in maintaining intestinal health. Soyabean curd is better than soyabean milk in taste and aroma, and resembles dairy curd. The curd is prepared by allowing the milk to cool, then seeded with a small quantity of cow's milk curd or soyabean milk curd and allowed to remain for 12 hours to set.

Taken regularly helps maintain intestinal health, prevent diseases arising from defective digestion and slows down the ageing process.

Soyabean is an important source of lecithin which is a very good natural emulsifier. Lecithin, as is well known, helps disperse deposits of fatty materials and cholesterol in certain vital organs[1]. It is rich in substances important for proper functioning of all living cells in the body. It is also an important component around brain and nerve cells. Lecithin is so abundant in soyabean that most lecithin used commercially comes from them.

Diabetes
Soyabean contains a fairly large amount of carbohydrate but little or no starch. It is, therefore, suitable for diabetic patients. The carbohydrate in it produces heat and energy without causing sugar to appear in the urine.

Skin Disorders
Soyabean is regarded as a valuable food remedy in eczema and other skin affections. It renders unnecessary the use of animal protein, that is, meat, eggs and milk and thus reduces the inflammatory activities in the skin and does not normally produce any sensitivity or allergic reactions which so frequently attend users of animal proteins. Liberal intake of soyabean reduces intense itching almost immediately and it disappears almost completely after a few days. The skin lesions also often vanish after a few days. Presumably lecithin content improves the skin health — a natural emulsifier which helps disperse fatty deposits and cholesterol.

Anaemia
Soyabean, being rich in iron, is beneficial in treating anaemia. However, since anaemic patients suffer from weak digestion, it should be given in light and easily digestable form.

Uses
Soyabeans are used as flour, green beans, sprouts and oil. Soya flour is one of the most widely used products of soyabean. It is by far

1. Dr. S.J. Singh, *Food Remedies*, pp. 188, Nature Cure Council of Medical Research, Lucknow, 1982.

more nutritious than the wheat flour. It contains 15 times as much calcium, seven times as much phosphorus, 10 times as much iron, 10 times as much thiamine and nine times as much riboflavin as wheat flour. In the West, soyabean flour industry has grown immensely. Soya flour is prepared by first roasting the soyabeans, removing their coating and then turning into powder.

Precautions: Soyabeans contain a bitter substance which can be removed by soaking soyabeans in six cupfuls of warm water containing half a teaspoon of sodium bicarbonate for 10 minutes. The process also removes the colouring matter from soyabean. Soyabeans contains a factor which inhibits the action of digestive enzyme trypsin. This factor can be destroyed by heating.[1]

SPINACH

Botanical Name: *Spinacia oleracea*
Indian Name: *Pālak*

Spinach is a high ranked green leafy vegetable with broad leaves. It is an annual winter crop which matures quickly. It has a round, very smooth and delicate stem. The leaves are alternate, succulent, fleshy, very smooth and dark green. They are generally five to eight cms long and one to one and half cms wide. The bottom of the leaf is shiny, with thick veins running across.

Origin and Distribution: Spinach is believed to have been first cultivated by the Arabs. The Persians cultivated it about 2,000 years ago. The Moors took it to Spain from where it spread to other parts of the world. The word spinach comes from a Spanish word *hispania.* In India it grows in abundance and thrives best in cool and moist climates. High humidity and cool temperature are conducive to rapid growth of its succulent, tender foliage.

1. Dr. Aman, Medicinal, *Secrets of Your Food*, pp. 142, Indo-American Hospital, Mysore, 1985.

Food Value: The chemical constituents of spinach are essential amino acids, iron, vitamin A and folic acid. It supplies the same amount of protein as one gets from an equal quantity of meat, fish, eggs and chicken. Other vegetables such as tomatoes, onions and cucumbers can be added to the raw tender spinach. With addition of a little lemon juice and olive oil it makes an excellent dish. The vitamin C content in lemon juice helps the body to absorb the entire amount of iron from the spinach consumed.

Spinach*

Food Value		Minerals and Vitamins	
Moisture	92.1%	Calcium	73 mg
Protein	2.0%	Phosphorus	21 mg
Fat	0.7%	Iron	10.9 mg
Minerals	1.7%	Vitamin C	28 mg
Fibre	0.6%	Small amounts of	
Carbohydrates	2.9%	Vitamin B Complex	
	100%		

**Values per 100 gms edible portion | Calorific Value - 17*

Natural Benefits and Curative Properties

The leaves of spinach are demulcent or soothing agents, refrigerant or coolants, diuretic and mildly laxative.

Constipation

Spinach juice cleans the digestive tract by removing any accumulated waste. It nourishes the intestines and tones up their movements. It is an excellent food remedy for constipation.

Anaemia

Spinach is a valuable source of high grade iron which promotes formation of haemoglobin and red blood cells. It is highly beneficial in preventing and treating anaemia.

Acidosis

Spinach is a rich source of calcium and other alkaline elements essential for keeping tissues clean and for preserving alkalinity of the blood. This helps prevent chronic diseases which thrive when too much acid is formed in the system.

Night Blindness

Spinach contains more vitamin A than most other green vegetables. This vitamin promotes health, especially health of the eyes. Lack of this vitamin may lead to night blindness. Spinach is thus an effective food remedy for preventing night blindness.

Tooth Disorders

Spinach juice is effective in strengthening the gums and · preventing and curing dental cavities. Chewing raw spinach leaves cures pyorrhoea. A mixture of carrot juice and spinach juice taken early in the morning can cure bleeding and ulcerated gums.

Pregnancy and Lactation

As one of the richest sources of folic acid, spinach is valuable during pregnancy and lactation. Megaloblastic anaemia of pregnancy occurs when the mother is deficient in folic acid. Folic acid deficiency occurs as it is required by the developing foetus. Regular use of spinach during pregnancy helps prevent deficiency of folic acid. It also prevents any potential abortion and accidental hemorrhage, deficient absorption of food associated with lassitude i.e. tiredness, shortness of breath, loss of weight and diarrhoea. Spinach is also a good source of nutrition for nursing or lactating mothers and improves the quality of their milk.

Urinary Disorders

Fresh spinach juice taken with tender coconut water once or twice a day acts as a very effective but safe diuretic with the combined action of both nitrates and potassium. It can be safely given in cystitis, nephritis and scanty urination caused by dehydration.

Respiratory Disorders

Infusion of fresh leaves spinach mixed with two teaspoonful of fenugreek seeds and a pinch of ammonium chloride and honey is an effective expectorant in treating bronchitis, tuberculosis, asthma and dry cough caused by throat congestion. It soothes the bronchioles, liquifies the tenacious sputum and forms healthy tissues in the lungs and increases resistance against respiratory infections. It should be taken in doses of 30 ml three times daily.

Uses

Spinach is often cooked as a green vegetable. It is also used in soups. Small, young and tender leaves of spinach can be used as raw salads. They are as appetising as tender lettuce leaves. The leaves of spinach are so juicy that no additional water is needed for cooking. The leaves should first be washed in several changes of water. The water which clings to the leaves is sufficient and no additional water is needed for cooking. The leaves should be cooked on moderate heat. It contributes roughage, colour and a bland flavour to the diet and it helps to balance the fuel foods in the menu.

Spinach however, contains a small amount of oxalic acid which is insoluble in the fluids of the alimentary tract and is harmful in gravels, gout and liver disease. Therefore, it should not be used by those suffering from these ailments.

TOMATO

Botanical Name: *Lycopersicon-esculentum*
Indian Name: *Tamātar*

Tomato is one of the most important vegetables. It is a short-lived perennial annual plant with extensive fibrous roots, solid, hairy stems and spirally arranged, mainly oval leaves. The fruit is a fleshy, round or lobed, smooth or furrowed, red, pink or yellow berry with numerous flat, slightly curved seeds.

Originally tomato was a small, wrinkled thick-skinned and seedy vegetable, much smaller in size and irregular in form. Scientific research has brought it to its present shape and quality. There now exist hundreds of varieties, many of which are smooth and globular, with almost solid pulp.

Origin and Distribution: Tomato is considered to be a native of South America, probably Peru-Equator. From there it was brought to Europe by the Spaniards in the 16th century. For several hundred years, it was grown as a garden ornament and called 'love apple'. In

1860, it was discovered that tomato was as good a food as any other fruit/vegetable. It is now grown in Malaysia, Indonesia, Philippines, tropical Africa, America and other tropical regions. It is second among the cultivated vegetables and is exceeded only by potato.

Food Value: Till about 170 years ago, tomato was considered poisonous. It was regarded by many as an acid-forming food which increased acidity in blood and body tissues. Because of this belief, those suffering from gout, rheumatism, arthritis and general acidosis were advised not to use it. It was also called a cancer-culprit. It was believed that it had no food value and supplied only colour and flavour to the diet. Later studies in nutritional chemistry, however, completely dispelled these baseless ideas. It is now considered to have unsurpassable nutritional and health-giving qualities.

Tomato*

Food Value		**Minerals and Vitamins**	
Moisture	94.0%	Calcium	48 mg
Protein	0.9%	Phosphorus	20 mg
Fat	0.2%	Iron	0.4 mg
Minerals	0.5%	Vitamin C	27 mg
Fibre	0.8%	Small amounts of	
Carbohydrates	3.4%	Vitamin B Complex	
	100%		

**Values per 100 gms edible portion | Calorific Value - 20*

Tomato is rich in calcium, phosphorus, vitamin C and carbohydrates. The carbohydrate in tomato is chiefly invert sugar which is the pre-digested form. It contains only a very small quantity of starch which is converted into sugar, chiefly dextrose, during the process of ripening.

Natural Benefits and Curative Properties

Tomato, is one of the most powerful deobstruent of the *Materia Medica*. It removes disease particles and opens natural channels of the body. It is a gentle natural stimulant for kidneys and helps to wash away disease causing toxins which contaminate our system. Tomatoes are at their best when fully ripe. The vitamin C content increases as they ripen. Tomato juice is probably one of the most widely used juices. Fresh, raw tomato juice is most beneficial and has an alkaline reaction when digested in concentrated form. External application of tomato is used as a cosmetic. Its pulp is applied liberally on the face and washed with warm water after about an hour. Repeated daily, it aids good complexion and removes pimples.

Acidosis

The tomato is essentially an alkaline vegetable. Its acid taste is due to the presence of about 0.5 per cent malic acid. It also contains 0.52 to 1.81 per cent citric acid and only a trace of oxalic acid. These acids in combination with sodium and potassium either form sodium or potassium acid malate, citrate or oxalate. Their end products, when oxidised in the body, are carbon dioxide, water and the carbonates of potassium and sodium. The latter has alkaline reaction. Tomatoes, thus leave an alkaline ash in the process of being oxidised by the body. This increases blood alkalinity, decreases urine and neutralises acid compounds such as phosphates, urea and ammonia, making tomatoes highly beneficial in treating acidosis and other diseases associated with too much acid in the system.

Diabetes

Because of its low carbohydrate contents, tomato is a very good food for diabetic patients and for those who want to reduce body weight. It is believed to be very effective in controlling the high percentage of sugar in urine of diabetic patients.

Eye Disorders

Being a rich source of vitamin A, tomatoes are a dependable preventive against night blindness, short sightedness and other eye diseases caused by the deficiency of the vitamin. Tomato leaves are useful in optic nerve and eye weakness. A small handful of freshly plucked tomato leaves should be covered with hot water for 15 minutes and then strained. A teaspoonful of this infusion taken three times daily before meals is a good tonic for eyes and optic nerve when taken three times daily before meals.

Obesity

Tomatoes are highly beneficial in treating obesity. One or two ripe tomatoes taken early morning before breakfast for a couple of months is considered a safe method of weight reduction; it also supplies essential food elements to preserve health.

Intestinal and Liver Disorders

A glassful of fresh tomato juice, mixed with a pinch of salt and pepper, taken early in the morning is considered an effective remedy for morning sickness, biliousness, sluggishness and diminished responsiveness of the liver, hepatitis and jaundice, indigestion, excessive formation of gas in the intestines, constipation, diarrhoea due to indigestion, burning in the gastrointestinal tract and constant burning sensation in the chest due to hiatus hernia, a condition in which a part of the stomach pushes up into the chest cavity.

Painful Joints

An oil prepared from the juice of the whole plant including leaves, mixed with equal quantity of *till-oil*, and heated until all water part evaporates massaged over painful joints and sprains and fomented with dry heat gives great relief. The oil can be preserved in bottles.

Respiratory Disorders

A glassful of fresh tomato juice mixed with honey and a pinch of powdered cardamom seeds, taken after swallowing three peeled cloves of garlic every night before going to bed, is considered highly beneficial in the treatment of tuberculosis and other lung infections. It increases resistance, prevents drug resistance and the relapse common in tubercular patients. In asthmatics, it reduces congestion in the bronchioles and checks hyper-secretion of mucous and reduces the spasms.

Urinary Disorder

Eating a tomato in the morning has been found to be an effective medicine for preventing formation of urinary calculi or stones. It is now known that deficiency of vitamins A and C and recurrent urinary tract infections are among the most important factors in formation of calculi. Tomatoes are rich in both vitamin A and C restrict the acid value of urine to 5.5 or less, thereby reducing the chances of infections by increasing acidity of the urine.

IMPORTANCE OF GRAIN CEREALS

Grains are generally classified as seeds of cereal plants. They are characterised by small size, hardness and low water content. Most grains belong to the family of grasses, scientifically known as gramineas.

The word cereal is derived from the name of Greek goddess of grains and harvests known as *Ceres*. Cereals have been a staple human diet from prehistoric times because of ease of their cultivation, good keeping qualities and great variety. Each of the cereals has unique properties and uses.

Cultivation of grains for human consumption (circa 10,000 BC) signified an era of stable civilisation in contrast to the earlier unsettled nomadic life. Ground cereals converted into bread evolved soon thereafter. Cereals have been modified and improved by centuries of cultivation and selective breeding.

There are numerous varieties of cereals; the most important being rice, wheat maize, millets, oats and barley.

Food Value: The whole grains of all cereals have a similar chemical composition and nutritive value. They are classified as carbohydrate-rich foods; the average carbohydrate content is 70 per cent per 100 gm. They provide energy and also some protein usually of good quality. The protein content of grains varies from 11.8 per cent for wheat to 8.5 per cent for rice per 100 gm. Whole cereals are good sources of calcium and iron but totally devoid of ascorbic acid and have very little of vitamin A activity. Yellow maize is the only cereal containing appreciable amounts of carotene. Whole grain cereals also contain significant amounts of B group vitamins. For a balanced diet, cereals should be supplemented by other proteins, minerals and vitamin A and C found in nuts, seeds, milk, fruits and green vegetables.

Whole grain cereals play an important role in our diet. Sprouted, they provide an increase in protein balance, as well as in all other nutrients, especially vitamin C. Complex form of their carbohydrate is a valuable source of fibre for the digestive process.

Natural Benefits and Curative Properties

All grains can be ground into flour for baking breads, cookies and cakes. In the earlier times freshly ground flour was used when fresh food was not easily available. This ensured that most nutrients in grains was retained. There is considerable loss of nutrients in mill-ground flour. When hulled, refined, ground, sterilised and bleached the grain becomes a grossly undernourished powder.

Wheat is by far the most popular flour; it there is a significant difference between whole wheat and plain white wheat flour. In the process of refining the whole wheat loses precious wheat germ, which is the very life of grain. The wheat germ contains the all important vitamin E. Grains are refined only to retain the endosperm for commercial use; the refined material appears cleaner, tastes better and is easier for baking bread, pastries and other confectioneries but products made from refined grain lack sufficient bulk and lead to numerous degenerative diseases and even cancer.

Four Essential Parts of Grains

1. the husk, hull or chaif, or the outer covering loosely attached to the grain,
2. the bran or the outer coat of the grain,
3. the germ or embryo, and
4. the endosperm which contains nutrients—considerable starch and small amounts of protein and fat.

BARLEY

Botanical Name: *Hordeum vulgars*
Indian Name: *Jau*

Barley is the fourth important cereal crop in the world and sixth in India. It is highly nutritious and an excellent body-builder. Although less palatable barley resembles wheat in composition. The barley grain, also called 'pearl barley', is prepared by removing its outer husk.

Origin and Distribution: Barely was the first cereal to be domesticated in the Middle East about 9,000 years ago and was probably the most important amongst the early cereals. Hulled barley was grown by the ancient Egyptians. It is now widely grown in Europe, arid regions near Sahara and the high plateau of Tibet. The world's largest producers of barley are the erstwhile Soviet regions, Germany, China and the United States.

Food Value: Barley is very nutritious and a rich source of protein and B-complex vitamins. Its protein quality is superior to that protein of corn and beans.

Most of the world's barley crop is converted into malt. It is most important grain used in the brewing of beer and much used in soups. Barley is also widely used as feed for live stock. However, it cannot be used for leavened bread because of low gluten content.

Barley*

Food Value		**Minerals and Vitamins**	
Moisture	12.5%	Calcium	26 mg
Protein	11.5%	Phosphorus	215 mg
Fat	1.3%	Iron	3 mg
Minerals	1.2%	Vitamin C	5 mg
Fibre	3.9%	Small amounts of	
Carbohydrates	69.6%	Vitamin B Complex	
	100%		

**Values per 100 gms edible portion | Calorific Value - 336*

Natural Benefits and Curative Properties

Barley has several medicinal virtues. Pearled barley grain is largely eaten as a food by invalids. The malt prepared from barley is used in the preparation of malt extract for using in the diet of infants and invalids.

Malt extract, which is more nutritious than the unmalted barley, is sourced from partially germinated and dried grain. Malt extract consists chiefly of dextrin and malt sugar and contains the ferment diastase enzyme which develops during the malting process. This ferment diastase possesses the power to convert starch into dextrin and sugar, thus assisting in digestion of starchy or farinaceous foods.[1]

Digestive System Disorders

Pearl barley has always been used in the Oriental traditional medicine for healing and rejuvenating the digestive system. A simple, yet effective folk remedy was to make a barley brew and sip it throughout the day, while restricting intake of other foods. This folk remedy has helped many and is used even to this day.

Barely brew is prepared by boiling one-quarter cup of all natural pearled barley in about 2.5 litres of water. When water has boiled down to about 1.25 litres, it is strained and the brew is ready. This all-natural barley brew helps digestive rejuvenation in two ways. It has a demulcent or soothing response and relieves the burning digestive actions. It also has a mucilaginous response and introduces a natural oily substance which helps to protect the abraded mucous membrane of the digestive system. Once the digestive system is soothed and healed, it promotes better assimilation of food.[2]

Fevers

The soothing properties barley are useful in fevers and all inflammatory conditions.

---

1. Dr. S.J. Singh, *Food Remedies*, pp. 43, Nature Cure Council of Medical Research, Lucknow, 1982.
2. Carlson Wade, *Health Secrets from the Orient*, pp. 59-60, Allied Publishers Private Lid., Bombay.

Urinary Disorders

Barley gruel with butter milk and lime juice is an excellent diuretic food. It is highly beneficial in treating urinary disorders, nephritis and cystitis.[1]

MAIZE

Botanical Name: *Zea manys*
Indian Name: *Makka*

After wheat and rice, maize is the world's most important cereal. The grains of maize are borne in separate inflorescences, which are completely enclosed as modified leaf sheaths or husks so that it is incapable of dispersing its sheets. The corn is at its best when it is well filled but soft and tender. The tender maize is chiefly liked for its high sugar content. It has more sugar than any other corn, hence its name — sweet corn.

Origin and Distribution: The name maize is derived from an Arawak-Carib word. 'mahiz'. It is this crop which made settled life possible for early civilisation in Mexico and Central America. Within a comparatively short time maize spread throughout the world and became an important source of carbohydrate food for developing and/or food scarce nations.

Maize*

Food Value		**Minerals and Vitamins**	
Moisture	14.9%	Calcium	10 mg
Protein	3.6%	Phosphorus	348 mg
Fat	1.5%	Iron	2 mg
Minerals	0.5%	Small amounts of	
Fibre	2.7%	Vitamin B Complex	
Carbohydrates	66.2%	and Vitamin E	
	100%		

**Values per 100 gms edible portion | Calorific Value - 342*

1. Dr. Aman, *Medicinal Secrets of Your Food*, pp. 527, Indo-American Hospital, Mysore, 1985.

Natural Benefits and Curative Properties

Bread made from the maize flour is nutritious, and digested without difficulty. Taken at intervals, this cereal helps to keep the colon clean. The dextrose produced from maize is used extensively in medicine.

Constipation

Popcorn made by heating the small grains is a wholesome and easily digested food. It has everything that the original grains have. It is not fattening and practically starch free; in the process of popping, the starch is converted into dextrine and intermediate carbohydrates, a digestive product, which is easily assimilable. It is a laxative and also provides bulk to faeces. It promotes peristalsis i.e. a series of muscle contractions in the digestive tract and is therefore a valuable food in constipation.

Uses

Maize is consumed in various ways. It is usually ground and pounded before consumption. The meal may be boiled, baked or fried. The whole grain can be boiled or roasted and or fermented. Maize meal can be cooked with water to provide a thick mush or dough. It can also be cooked with water to provide gruel, porridge or soup. Cornbread is made by mixing the meal with wheat flour. Immature cobs, preferably of sweet corn, are boiled and eaten as corn on its cob or the grain may be removed and eaten as a vegetable, or may be canned. More mature cobs are roasted.

RICE

Botanical Name: *Orya Sativa*
Indian Name: *Chawal*

Rice is a much-revered oriental food and perhaps the most important tropical cereal. It is a staple food of about half the human race and is often the main source of calories.

Origin and Distribution: One of the earliest mention of rice dates back to 2800 BC, when a Chinese emperor established a ceremonial protocol for the planting rice which was used by the royal physicians for healing purposes. It was grown in India as far back as in 3000 BC, when it appeared as a plant called 'Newaree'. By general consensus rice was domesticated in India or Indo-china. Enormous quantities of rice are now grown in India and Asia.

Food Value: Starch constitutes bulk of the rice grain. The protein content of rice is lower than that of wheat, but of superior quality and utilised better by the body than the wheat protein.

Ancient and modern Oriental healers have always advocated using natural brown rice as a key to youthful health; milling removes many of the valuable B-complex vitamins and some of the minerals.

Natural Benefits and Curative Properties

In the Eastern countries rice has always been considered a magical healer. It was originally believed to have medicinal values that

Raw Handpounded Rice*

Food Value		**Minerals and Vitamins**	
Moisture	13.3%	Calcium	10 mg
Protein	7.5%	Phosphorus	190 mg
Fat	1.0%	Iron	3.2 mg
Minerals	0.9%	Small amounts of	
Fibre	0.6%	Vitamin B Complex	
Carbohydrates	76.7%		
	100%		

Calorific Value - 346

Raw Milled Rice*

Food Value		**Minerals and Vitamins**	
Moisture	13.7%	Calcium	10 mg
Protein	6.8%	Phosphorus	160 mg
Fat	0.5%	Iron	3.1 mg
Minerals	0.6%	Small amounts of	
Fibre	0.2%	Vitamin B Complex	
Carbohydrates	78.2%		
	100%		

**Values per 100 gms edible portion | Calorific Value - 345*

could restore tranquility and peace to those easily upset. It has been mentioned in early Oriental writings that natural whole grain brown rice is a perfect healing food. In the ancient literature of Thailand, Mynamar, Malaysia and Indo-China rice is mentioned as a source of health. It was also revered as a food of divine health and used in religious offerings.

Modern researches have confirmed the belief of that eating brown rice is a source of serenity and tranquility. It contains all elements needed for maintaining good health.

Rice is about 98 per cent digestible. It is one of the most easily and quickly digested of all foods — it gets fully digested in about one hour. Rice starch is different from other grain starches; it contains 100 per cent amylopectin which is amongst the most completely and rapidly digested grain starch. This makes rice an ideal health food for those who seek speedy and healthy assimilation.

Internal Rejuvenation

Rice protein, which comprises upto eight per cent of the grain, has a special benefit; it has eight of the essential amino acids in a

Types of Rice

Brown Rice: Rice from which only the husk has been removed but layers of bran and most of the germ retained.

Milled Rice or White Rice: Rice from which husk, germ and bran layers have almost fully been removed by machine.

Hand Pounded Rice: Rice from which husk, germ and bran layers have been partly removed without machinery.

Polished Rice: Rice milled to a high degree and then coated with some foreign substance such as glucose or talcum.

Parboiled Rice: Paddy processed by steaming or soaking in water, heated and dried, and then milled or hand pounded.

delicately balanced proportions. A complete internal rejuvenation takes place when rice protein is metabolised into health-building amino acids. These amino acids build resilient muscles, healthy skin and hair, clearer eyesight and nourish the heart, lungs, tendons and ligaments, brain, nervous system and glandular network.

The B-complex vitamins, especially thiamin, riboflavin and niacin offered by natural brown rice promote youthful energy and nourishment to skin and blood vessels. An abundance of minerals in natural brown rice help nourish the hormonal system, heal wounds and regulate blood pressure. Rice also contains iron to enrich the bloodstream, and phosphorus and potassium to maintain internal water balance along with other nutrients.

High Blood Pressure/Hypertension

Rice has a low-fat, low-cholesterol and low-salt content. It makes a perfect diet for hypertensive persons who are advised salt-restricted diets. Researchers note that wherever rice is the main food, there is a corresponding benefit of youthful vitality and a low rate of hypertension. Calcium in brown rice, in particular, soothes and relaxes the nervous system and helps relieve symptoms of high blood pressure.

Body Balance

Rice diet, in combination with milk, creates a marvellous body balance. In this regimen, natural brown rice is used as the only solid food throughout the day. Fresh milk is taken with each rice meal. The rice may be cooked in any manner but without salt. The milk should be cool but not cold. The nutrients in rice form a unique balance with those in milk. The two notable amino acids, isoleucine and lysine, in the milk are greatly strengthened by rice protein, thereby forming stronger body-building blocks. The natural lactic acid in milk works with rice protein to aid absorption of iron.

Digestive Disorders

Rice has a very low fibre content and therefore extremely soothing to the digestive system. This makes it an ideal for digestive system disorders. Thick gruel of rice mixed with a glassful of buttermilk and a ripe banana given twice a day is a highly nutritious in typhoid, gastric ulcer, gastritis, stomach and intestinal cancer, colitis, diarrhoea, dysentery, piles, rectal fissure, indigestion, and in acute febrile diseases related to fever, hepatitis or inflammation of liver, jaundice, morning sickness, acute dilatation of the stomach, burning and indigestion due to hiatus hernia, excessive accumulation of the gas in the intestines, and all diseases where a mild and light diet is indicated.

Diarrhoea in Children

A teaspoonful of powder of charred par-boiled rice mixed with a glassful of butter-milk given in doses of one tablespoon every half an hour brings excellent results.

Skin Inflammation

Rice flour, dusted thickly has a cooling and soothing effect in small-pox, measles, prickly heat and other inflammatory affections of the skin including burns and scalds. It allays heat and irritation. Rice powder should be used soon after the occurrence of injury in case of burns and scalds and should be dusted thickly over the affected surface.

Uses

Rice is usually cooked by boiling in water or by steaming, and is eaten mostly with pulses, vegetables, fish or meat. There are two varieties of rice, the long grain rice and the short and medium grain rice. When cooked, grains of the long variety soften but do not stick to each other. This variety is especially good for consuming with curries, stews or as a side dish with a sauce or gravy. Short and medium varieties have short, plump grains which cook tender and moist, with the particles tending to cling together. They are especially good for preparing puddings.

WHEAT

Botanical Name: *Triticum sativum*
Indian Name: *Gehun*

Wheat is one of the most valuable of all cereals and a good source of energy. With its coating of bran, vitamins and minerals, it is an excellent health-building food.

Origin and Distribution: Wild species of wheat have been reported from the archaeological site of Tell Mureybal on the banks of the Euphrates, circa 800 BC, and at Ali Kosh in south-west Iran (7500-6750 BC). Species of wheat appeared in India, probably before the fourth millennium BC, and in China sometime before the beginning of the Christian era. India now ranks fourth among the wheat producing countries.

Food Value: Because of quality and quantity of its characteristic protein called gluten wheat is the principal cereal used for bread making. It is gluten that makes bread dough stick and gives it the ability to retain gas; the higher the proportion of gluten in the flour, better it is for making leavened bread. The germ or embryo of the wheat is relatively rich in protein, fat and several of the B vitamins. So is the scutellum in wheat, which contains 50 times more thiamin than the whole grain. The outer layers of the endosperm and the aleurone contain a higher concentration of protein, vitamins and phytic acid than the inner endosperm. The inner endosperm contains most of the starch and protein in the grain.

Wheat is usually ground into flour before use. In ancient times wheat grains were crushed between two large stones. This method of stone-grinding preserved all parts of the kernel and the product was called 'whole wheat'. Once finely ground, it becomes whole wheat flour. Stone ground wheat is more nutritious than mill ground wheat; the grain is ground slowly, remains unheated, and a whole food. The modern roller mills grind wheat hundreds times

Whole Wheat Flour*

Food Value		Minerals and Vitamins	
Moisture	12.2%	Calcium	48 mg
Protein	12.1%	Phosphorus	355 mg
Fat	1.7%	Iron	11.5 mg
Minerals	2.7%	Small amounts of	
Fibre	1.9%	Vitamin B Complex	
Carbohydrates	69.4%		
	100%		

Calorific Value - 341

Refined Wheat Flour*

Food Value		Minerals and Vitamins	
Moisture	13.3%	Calcium	23 mg
Protein	11.0%	Phosphorus	12.1 mg
Fat	0.9%	Iron	2.5 mg
Minerals	0.6%	Small amounts of	
Fibre	0.3%	Vitamin B Complex	
Carbohydrates	73.9%		
	100%		

**Values per 100 gms edible portion | Calorific Value - 348*

faster, but impoverish it by removing the wheat germ, resulting in colossal loss in vitamins and minerals in the process.

Natural Benefits and Curative Properties

Wheat in its natural form contains several medicinal virtues. Every part of the whole wheat grain supplies elements needed by the human body. Starch and gluten in wheat provide heat and energy; the inner bran coats provide phosphates and other mineral salts; the outer bran, the much-needed roughage; the germ provides vitamins B and E; and protein of wheat helps build and repair muscule tissue. The wheat germ, which is removed in the process of refining, is also rich in essential vitamin E, the lack of which can lead to heart disease. The loss of vitamins and minerals in the refined wheat flour has led to widespread constipation and other digestive problems and nutritional disorders. The whole wheat, which includes bran and wheat germ, therefore, provides protection against diseases such as constipation, ischaemic heart disease, disease of the colon called diverticulum, appendicitis, obesity and diabetes.

Dr. Ann Wigmore, founder-director of the Hippocrates Health Institute, Boston, U.S.A., is one of the proponents of the 'wheat grass therapy'. According to her, 'guided by spiritual mentality and nourished only by live uncooked food, the body will run indefinitely, unhampered by sickness'. Dr. Wigmore utilises the chlorophyll present in wheat grass as a body cleanser, rebuilder and neutraliser of toxins.[1] Wheat grass juice provides the body with vital nourishment and extra energy. This juice contains nearly 70 per cent chlorophyll. It is also a rich source of vitamin A, B and C. Besides it contains minerals like calcium, iron, magnesium, phosphorus, potassium, sodium, sulphur, cobalt and zinc.

Chlorophyll, one of the main constituents of wheat grass is very beneficial for the body; with its high vitamin and mineral content chlorophyll purifies the blood. This helps by the body to cleanse and rebuild itself. Drinking this juice regularly neutralises toxins thus helping to maintain good health.

Tooth Disorders

Wheat is valuable in preventing and curing pyorrhoea. It takes longer to eat wheat and it is generally eaten along with other foods; it compels the chewing of other foods also. This not only exercises the teeth and gums but also aids digestion.

Wheat grass juice is an excellent mouth wash for sore throats and pyorrhoea. It also prevents tooth decay and tooth aches. It is beneficial to chew wheat grass; it draws out toxins from the gums and checks bacterial growth.

Constipation

Wheat bran, which is generally discarded in milling, is more wholesome and nourishing than the flour itself. It is an excellent laxative. The laxative effects of bran are much superior to those of fruits or green vegetables; the cellulose of bran is more easily broken down by bacteria while passing through the intestine.[2] The bran

1. Dr. Ann Wigmore, *Be your Own Doctor*, pp. 5, Flemisphere Press inc, New York.
2. Dr. S.J. Singh, *Food Remedies*, pp. 211, Nature Cure Council of Medical Research, Lucknow, 1982.

contains rich concentration of cellulose which forms a bulk-mass in the intestines and helps increased peristalsis and better evacuation.

Skin Diseases

It has been scientifically proved that chlorophyll arrests growth and development of harmful bacteria. Wheat grass therapy can be effectively used for skin diseases and ulcerated wounds; it retards bacterial action, promotes cell activity and normal re-growth. Regular drinking of wheat grass juice creates an unfavourable environment for bacterial growth. Poultice of wheat grass juice can be applied on the infected area as a natural sterilizer.

> Forget about nuclear war; the real weapons of mass destruction are fast food, highly processed carbs, and refined sugar!
>
> Brian Quebbemann, M.D.

Externally, wheat flour is useful as a dusting powder over inflamed surface as in burns, scalds and various itching and burning eruptions. Whole wheat flour, mixed with vinegar, boiled and applied outwardly removes freckles.[1]

Digestive System Disorders

As an enema wheat grass juice helps detoxify the walls of colon. The general procedure is to give an enema with lukewarm or neem water. After waiting for 20 minutes, 90 to 120 ml of wheat grass juice enema is given which should be retained for 15 minutes. This enema is very helpful in disorders of the colon, mucous and ulcerative colitis, chronic constipation and bleeding piles.[2]

Circulatory Disorders

The chlorophyll content of wheat grass enhances heart and lung functions. Capillary activity also increases while toxaemia or blood

---

1. Ibid, p. 209
2. Dr. T. Chandrashekar, *Wheat Grass Juice*, Health Herald, Ban'lore, Jan '86, p. 11.

poisoning is reduced. Due to increased iron content in the blood and haemoglobin, lungs function better, oxygenation improves and the effect of carbon-dioxide is minimised. It is for this reason that wheat grass juice is prescribed for circulatory disorders.

Wheat grass is grown by soaking a good variety of wheat for eight to 10 hours. The water is then drained and grains allowed to sprout for 15 hours. Earthen pots or wooden trays can be used to grow wheat grass. These trays should be filled with compost manure. Wheat sprouts should be spread and the trays kept away from sunlight in a room. The trays should be sprinkled with water once or twice a day and allowed to remain for six to seven days until the grass grows about 15 cms high.

Chewing wheat grass is the easiest method to benefit from it. As an alternative to chewing, wheat grass can be cut finely and ground in a grinder with water added to extract wheat grass juice. This juice should be taken within 10 to 15 minutes after extraction. In the early stages of wheat grass therapy about 100 ml to 150 ml of wheat grass juice is advised daily. As the body becomes accustomed to its taste, the quantity of juice can be gradually increased to about 250 ml to 300 ml per day. Wheat grass juice should be mixed thoroughly with saliva before being swallowed slowly. The juice should be taken an hour before a meal or two to three hours after the meal.

Uses

Chappatis made from whole wheat flour called *atta* are the commonest form in which wheat is eaten in India, Pakistan and Iran. Shredded wheat called *dalia* is wholesome and equally popular. It is cooked by soaking two tablespoonful of crushed or shredded wheat for half an hour and then cooking it on a slow fire till the water nearly dries up. Thereafter milk and honey may be added to taste. It is a nourishing morning breakfast food item.

Pulses and Legumes
Natural Benefits and Curative Properties

Include pulses and legumes in your meals for a healthier life.

Nutritive properties of pulses are quite similar to those of whole cereal grains but with several important differences.

1. Pulse protein is low in sulphur containing amino acids, but rich in lysine[1] in which many cereals are deficient. A combination of pulses and cereal proteins may, therefore, have a nutritive value as good as animal proteins.
2. As a class, pulses are good sources of the B group vitamins except riboflavin. More important, the greater part of these vitamins present in the harvested seeds is actually consumed. There are no losses comparable with those that those that take place in the milling and cooking of cereals. Pulses are therefore, an excellent preventive against beriberi.
3. Although pulses are devoid of vitamin C, large amounts of ascorbic acid are formed on germination. Sprouted pulses therefore become an important food which protects against scurvy.
4. Some legumes have a good fibre and are therefore good for diabetics, especially type 1 and 2.

1. An essential amino acid which cannot be synthesised in the body. It inhibits proliferation of viruses & therefore protective.

IMPORTANCE OF PULSES

Pulses are dried edible seeds of cultivated legumes belonging to the family of peas, beans and lentils. The word pulse is taken from the Latin *puls*, meaning pottage or thick pap. Pulses are a large family and various species are capable or surviving in very different climates and soils.

Pulses are cultivated throughout the world and occupy an important place in human diet. However, they make a more important contribution to the Eastern diet than to the Western diet. The vegetarians, especially in India, depend largely on cereals and pulses for dietary protein and energy.

Food Value: Pulses contain more protein than any other plant. They serve as a low-cost source of protein to meet the needs of a large section of the population and have often been justifiably described as 'poor man's meat'. Their low moisture content and hard testa or seed-coat permits storage over long time periods. In addition to providing dry pulses, many of the crops are grown for their edible green pods and unripe seeds. Nutritionally, immature fruits have distinctly different properties than those of the mature seeds; the protein content is lower but they are relatively richer in vitamins and soluble carbohydrates. The leaves and shoots of some of the crops are used as pot-herbs.

In general, pulses contain 20 to 28 per cent protein per 100 gm with the exception of soyabean which has as much as 47 per cent protein. Their carbohydrate content is about 60 per cent per 100 gm while soyabean has about 30 per cent. Pulses are also fairly good sources of thiamin and niacin and provide calcium, phosphorus and iron. On an average 100 gm of pulses contain energy 345 kcal, 24.5 gm protein, 140 mg calcium, 300 mg phosphorus, 8 mg iron, 0.5 mg thiamin, 0.3 mg riboflavin. and 2 mg niacin.

Uses

Pulses are used in various forms. Pulses, dehusked, decorticated and whole seed, are used as *dhal* taken with *chappatis* and/or rice. Whole seeds take longer to cook than the dehusked and decorticated ones which are relatively better digestible.

The digestion of pulses and the absorption of their principal nutrients is practically complete and nearly as effective as the assimilation of cereals. However, only small quantities of well-cooked pulses should be included in the diets of patients with stomach disorders.

Pulses are also widely used or mixed in flour such as that of Bengal gram, green gram, black gram, known as 'besan'. It is used for mixing with cereal flour for *chappatis* and other preparations.

The practice of utilizing germinated seed or sprouted pulses or young seedlings of pulses as a fresh vegetable is widespread in South Asia. Storing of dried seed and sprouting them later, as and when required, enables a continuous supply of fresh vegetable material to be produced. There is an amazing increase in nutrients in sprouted pulses when compared to their dried embryo. In the process of sprouting, the vitamins, minerals and protein increase substantially with corresponding decrease in calories and carbohydrate content.

Sprouting of pulses not only improves their nutritive value but also digestibility. During sprouting starch is broken down to dextrin and maltose, and proteins are broken down to polypeptides, peptides and amino acids. Some of the bound iron is converted to a more readily assimilable form. Phosphorus is liberated from phytate. The ascorbic acid or vitamin C content rises from negligible levels in the seed to 12 mgs per 100 gms after 48 hours of germination. Riboflavin and niacin content also increase significantly. These changes are caused by enzymes which become active during germination.

BENGAL GRAM

Botanical Name: *Cicer arietinum*
Indian Name: *Channā*

Bengal gram or chickpeas is one of the most important pulses in India. There are many varieties of chickpeas which are used to cooking including *dhal*, hummus, curries and snacks. Kala chana or Bengal gram is a smaller and darker variety of chickpeas which is equally popular.

Kala chana looks like dried, shrivelled, dark brown mini versions of chickpeas. The outer shell of this legume is removed and the remaining product split to make chana *dhal* or split chickpeas.

Origin and Distribution: Bengal gram is said to have originated in west Asia and then spread to India and Europe. The crop was also known to the ancient Egyptians, Hebrews and the Greeks.

Food Value: The whole dried Bengal gram seeds are cooked or boiled. They are also consumed raw after soaking in water. For preparing *dhal*, the seeds are sprinkled with water overnight to soften the husk and then dried before milling. Flour is made by grinding the seeds. This flour is one of the main ingredients of many forms of Indian confectionary made with ghee and sugar. It is also used for preparing many tasty snacks like *sev*, *chila*, *pakoras* and curries like *koftas*. Green pods and tender shoots are used as a vegetable.

Natural Benefits and Curative Properties

Bengal gram has many medicinal properties. Soaked overnight in water and chewed with honey it acts as a general tonic. The liquid, obtained by soaking the seeds and then macerating them, is also a tonic. Sprouted Bengal gram is rich in B-complex and C vitamins. Cooked germinated gram is a wholesome food for children and invalids. However, excessive use of Bengal gram can cause indigestion and can precipitate urinary calcium due to high concentration of oxalic acid and urinary stone or calculi.

Bengal Gram (Whole Dried Seeds)*

Food Value		Minerals and Vitamins	
Moisture	9.8%	Calcium	202 mg
Protein	17.1%	Phosphorus	312 mg
Fat	5.3%	Iron	10.2 mg
Minerals	3.0%	Vitamin C	3 mg
Fibre	3.9%	Small amounts of	
Carbohydrates	60.9%	Vitamin B Complex	
	100%		

Calorific Value - 360

Bengal Gram (dhal made from Seeds)*

Food Value		Minerals and Vitamins	
Moisture	9.9%	Calcium	56 mg
Protein	20.8%	Phosphorus	331 mg
Fat	5.6%	Iron	9.1 mg
Minerals	2.7%	Vitamin C	1 mg
Fibre	1.2%	Small amounts of	
Carbohydrates	59.8%	Vitamin B Complex	
	100%		

**Values per 100 gms edible portion | Calorific Value - 372*

Diabetes

Experiments have shown that the intake of water extract of Bengal gram enhances the utilization of glucose in both diabetic and normal persons. Tests were conducted at CFTRI* Laboratories, Mysore, on a chronic diabetic patients whose insulin requirement was of the order of 40 units a day. When kept on a diet which included liberal supplements of Bengal gram extract, the condition improved considerably and the patients' insulin requirement reduced to about 20 units per day. Diabetic patients on a prescribed diet which did not severely restrict their intake of carbohydrates, but included liberal amounts of Bengal gram extract, also showed considerable improvement in fasting blood sugar levels, glucose tolerance, urinary excretion of sugar and general condition.

Anaemia

Fresh juice of Bengal gram leaves is rich in iron and highly beneficial in treating of iron deficiency anaemias. A tablespoonful of fresh juice mixed with honey is advised for this condition.

* Central Food Technology Research Institute

Painful Menstruation

A bath prepared by putting the entire Bengal gram plant in hot water is highly beneficial in painful menstruation. It may be taken in the form of a sitting steam bath.

Skin and Hair Disease

Flour of unroasted Bengal gram is an effective cleansing agent and used regularly acts as a cosmetic skin bleach. In allergic skin diseases like eczema, contact dermatitis, scabies, washing the skin with this flour is highly beneficial. Bengal gram flour mixed with curd is used to prepare a paste which is applied to the face and washed off after some time; this is a traditional treatment of pimples. Washing the hair with Bengal gram flour keeps them clean, soft and disease free.

Sexual Dysfunction

Flour of the puffed Bengal gram is a highly nutritive and an effective remedy for impotency and premature ejaculation. For better results, two tablespoonful of this flour mixed with sugar, powdered dates and skimmed milk powder is packed in airtight container and used when required.

BLACK GRAM

Botanical Name: *Phasleolus mungo*
Indian Name: *Urad*

Black gram is one of the most prized pulses of India. It is an erect, sub-erect or trailing, hairy annual herb. It is one of the most nutritious pulses.

Origin and Distribution: Black gram originated in ancient India. It was later introduced elsewhere by Indian immigrants. It now cultivated throughout Asia and in Africa but nowhere is it as important as in India.

Food Value: Black gram is boiled and eaten whole or after splitting into *dhal*. It is extensively used in various culinary preparations like idli, curries and papad. The green pods eaten as a vegetable are highly nutritious. The hulls or the outer covering of gram and straw are used as cattle feed.

Black Gram*

Food Value		**Minerals and Vitamins**	
Moisture	10.9%	Calcium	154 mg
Protein	24.0%	Phosphorus	385 mg
Fat	1.4%	Iron	9.1 mg
Minerals	3.2%	Small amounts of	
Fibre	0.9%	Vitamin B Complex	
Carbohydrates	59.6%		
	100%		

**Values per 100 gms edible portion | Calorific Value - 347*

Natural Benefits and Curative Properties

Black gram is demulcent or a soothing and a cooling agent. It is an aphrodisiac and nervine tonic. However, excessive use of black gram may cause flatulence which can be prevented by adding a little asafoetida, pepper and ginger in the culinary preparations. It should not be taken by those predisposed to rheumatic diseases and urinary calculi as it contains a high concentration of oxalic acid.

Diabetes

Germinated black gram taken with half a cupful of fresh bitter gourd juice and a teaspoonful of honey is highly beneficial in treating mild diabetes. It should be used once daily for three to four months with restricted carbohydrate diet. Even in severe cases, regular use of this combination, with other precautions, is useful in preventing complications due to malnutrition in diabetic patients.

Sexual Dysfunction

Black gram *dhal* soaked in water for about six hours and fried in cow's ghee, after draining the water is an excellent sex tonic. It can be used with wheat bread and honey in functional impotency, premature ejaculation and thin semen.

Nervous Disorders

Eaten with half boiled egg the above preparation is an excellent tonic in disorders related to the nervous system like nerve weakness, weak memory, schizophrenia and hysteria.

Hair Disorders
Washing hair with a paste of cooked black gram *dhal* and fenugreek lengthens the hair, keeps them black and cures dandruff.

Digestive Disorders
Black gram is valuable in digestive system disorders. In the form of a decoction it is useful in dyspepsia, gastric catarrh, dysentery and diarrhoea.

Rheumatism/Rheumatic Afflictions
A liniment made from black gram is useful as an external application in rheumatism, contracted knee and stiff shoulder. It is prepared by boiling about 4 kgs of black gram pulse in approximately in 38 litres of water. Once boiled down to about 10 litres and strained, the decoction is boiled with about 2.5 litres of sesame oil and ½ kg of rock salt till the water evaporates. Paste of the fresh root is also useful in rheumatic pains.

GREEN GRAM

Botanical Name: *Phaseolus aureus*
Indian Name: *Mung*

Green gram is one of the most wholesome pulses in India. It does not create any bloating or heaviness or flatulence associated with other pulses.

Origin and Distribution: This plant is a native of India and has been in cultivation since the ancient times. It was introduced early into Southern China, Indo-China and Java and later into East and Central Africa, the West Indies and the United States.

Food Value: Green gram is highly nutritious. It is consumed in the form of whole dried seeds and as *dhal*, prepared by splitting the seeds in a mill. After sprouting the mung beans become even more nutritious. The beans are soaked overnight, drained and placed in a dark room where they are sprinkled with water every few hours.

The sprouts are ready in about three days. About half a kilo of dry beans gives about 3.5 kgs of sprouts. There is an amazing increase in nutrients in sprouted beans when compared to their dried embryo.

Green Gram (Whole dried Seeds)*

Food Value		Minerals and Vitamins	
Moisture	10.4%	Calcium	124 mg
Protein	24.0%	Phosphorus	326 mg
Fat	1.3%	Iron	7.3 mg
Minerals	3.5%	Small amounts of	
Fibre	4.1%	Vitamin B Complex	
Carbohydrates	56.7%		
	100%		

Calorific Value - 334

Green Gram (*Dhal*)*

Food Value		Minerals and Vitamins	
Moisture	10.1%	Calcium	75 mg
Protein	24.5%	Phosphorus	405 mg
Fat	1.2%	Iron	8.5 mg
Minerals	3.5%	Small amounts of	
Fibre	0.8%	Vitamin B Complex	
Carbohydrates	59.9%		
	100%		

**Values per 100 gms edible portion | Calorific Value - 348*

Natural Benefits and Curative Properties

Cooked *dhal* of green gram is a digestive food and widely used in the diet of those recuperating from illness. Its regular use during childhood, pregnancy and lactation helps get the required nutrition and promotes health. It is an aperient i.e. a laxative, when given in large quantities. The soup made from green gram is highly nutritious.

Applied in the form of powder, green gram is said to be useful in relieving heat or burning of the eyes. A poultice of this powder is useful for checking secretion of milk and reducing distention of mammary glands.

Fevers

Water in which green gram has been soaked makes an excellent remedy for cholera, measles, chicken-pox, small-pox, typhoid and all types of fevers. It can be given in a small quantity even during acute phase of appendicitis.

Beauty Aid
Flour of the green gram is an excellent detergent and can be used as a substitute for soap. It removes the dirt and does not cause any skin irritation. It makes a good facial bleach and improves complexion. Black gram flour with green gram paste is also used as a hair wash to lengthen hair and prevent dandruff.

Uses
Dried beans are boiled and eaten either whole or after splitting into *dhal*. They are parched and ground into flour after removing the testa or the seed-coat. This flour is used in various Indian and Chinese dishes. The green pods are eaten as a sprouted vegetable.

PIGEON PEA

Botanical Name: *Cajanus cajan*
Indian Name: *Arhar*

Pigeon pea is an important pulse. It is a woody, short-lived perennial shrub. The fruit is a flattened pod. Seeds vary in size, shape and colour, are usually round or oval, white or greyish, red, brown purplish or speckled, with a small white hilium.

Origin and Distribution: Pigeon pea is probably a native of tropical Africa; its seeds have also been found in Egyptain tombs and is assumed that it was cultivated there before 2000 BC. Pigeon peas were also cultivated in Madagascar and now has the greatest number of varieties. Pigeon peas are now spread throughout tropics and subtropics. The areas of cultivation include India, Malaysia, Indonesia, Philippines, the Caribbean, East and West Africa.

Food Value: The fresh leaves are used as a vegetable. The immature pods are also cooked. Dried seeds are added to soups and stews. The ripe dry seeds are boiled and eaten as a pulse. In India these are split into *dhal* and the dried husks, seeds and broken *dhal* are used as cattle feed.

Pigeon Pea*

Food Value		Minerals and Vitamins	
Moisture	13.4%	Calcium	73 mg
Protein	22.3%	Phosphorus	304 mg
Fat	1.7%	Iron	5.8 mg
Minerals	3.5%	Small amounts of Vitamin B Complex	
Fibre	1.5%		
Carbohydrates	57.6%		
	100%		

**Values per 100 gms edible portion | Calorific Value - 335*

Natural Benefits and Curative Properties

Pigeon pea is easily digested, has several medicinal properties and suitable for those recovering from illness. It relieves inflammation of internal organs. However, excessive use of pigeon pea may causes hyper-acidity and wind in the intestines. It is therefore, to be avoided in cases of gastric ulcer and heart disease.

Baldness

Applied regularly a fine paste made of this pulse is highly useful in bald patches.

Hepatitis/Jaundice

The expressed juice of the leaves with a little salt is highly beneficial in the treatment of jaundice. 60ml of this juice is advised daily.

Checking Breast Milk Secretion

The pulse and leaves ground into a paste, warmed and applied over the mamma has the effect of checking the secretion of breast milk.

Inflammation

Leaves of the plant are effective in all inflammatory conditions. A poultice made with the seeds also reduces swelling.

Piles

Paste of the leaves mixed with a teaspoonful of paste of neem leaves is highly beneficial in treating piles and itching in the anus. It should be taken once daily for a week.

IMPORTANCE OF NUTS AND SEEDS

Nuts and seeds are perhaps the most potent of all foods. Nuts are the seeds from which plant life grows provided seeds remain in the ground until germination. Seeds have always been symbols of resurrection; they contain the embryo, the reproductive power which is of vital importance for the lives of human beings and their health. Dry, hard and tough — seeds appear lifeless but given moisture and soil, they sprout and produce not one but many more seeds or nuts.

There are a variety of nuts. The most popular among them are almond, cashewnut, coconut, groundnut, pistachio and walnut. All varieties contain concentrated high nutritional value.

Nut Butter

Nut butter is excellent to optimise nutritive benefits of nuts. It can be prepared at home by removing the skin of nuts and then grinding them into a fine paste.

This butter can be put on fruits for added protein, in dressings and added to soups or used in vegetables. The butter is easily digested and especially beneficial for the elderly who may not like meat or cannot eat because of dental issues. The B vitamins, minerals and proteins in the butter act to improve the appetite. However unheated and unsalted nut butter should be used.

Food Value: Seeds provide important nutrients needed for growth. They are excellent sources of protein and essential unsaturated fatty acids. They are also amongst the best natural sources of lecithin, most B-complex vitamins and vitamin E, all of which are important elements for preservation of health and prevention of premature ageing. Besides, they are rich sources of minerals and fibre.

Similarly, nuts are high in protein, fat and carbohydrates. They are rich in several minerals such as potassium, the healer; sodium, the preserver of youth; calcium and phosphorus which are essential for strong, bones and teeth; and sulphur which purifies and activates the body. Raw nuts are generously supplied with B vitamins, which are valuable for the brain and the nervous system as well as vitamin F which is needed for all round development. Some seeds and nuts also contain vitamin A and C. The general composition, per 100 gms, is roughly formed by 10 to 25 per cent protein, 40 to 60 per cent fat, 10 to 20 per cent carbohydrates, three to five per cent cellulose and nearly two per cent minerals.

Nut Milk

Nut milk is the most easily digested form of nuts. It makes rich non-acid-forming drinks, full of nourishment. Nut milk is prepared from blanched nuts soaked in water for a few hours to soften the structure of the kernel. Then 90 gm of soaked nuts are put in 150 ml of water and kept for two or three minutes in a liquefier and flavoured with honey or any fruit concentrate. The fluid resembles dairy milk in composition and appearance. It is so easily digested that it can be used in baby feed. Almond milk is a rich alkaline drink, high in protein and easy to assimilate and absorb.

Nut milk can also be used as a sherbet by adding sugar and lime juice. The milk may be curdled like dairy milk with the addition of a little curd.

Natural Benefits and Curative Properties

Seeds contain pacifarins, an antibiotic resistance factor, which increases our natural resistance to disease. They also contain auxones, natural substances which help produce vitamins in the body and play an important role in rejuvenating cells, thereby preventing premature ageing.

Sprouted seeds are valuable sources of protein, vitamins and complex carbohydrates. Germination of seeds increases their nutritional value enormously. All seeds should ideally be eaten raw but those which can be sprouted, should be sprouted for maximum nutrition.

Nuts should be used in their natural raw state. Raw nuts are among the foods with highest fat content. But the fat of nuts is completely natural and unprocessed and is best for body. It is especially rich in linoleic acid and is least damaging to the heart and arteries.

Nuts often produce oil half their weight. The high energy value of the nuts is mainly due to their oil content. They provide approximately 600 calories per 100 gms compared to 348 for wheat, 346 for lentils, and 283 for dates of equal weight. Nut oil is used for cooking. Pure nut oils are often used in medicine.

Raw nuts are a safe food; their hard shell offer an effective barrier against bacteria. They can be preserved with all nutrition intact for long periods in their natural unshelled state. Being extremely low in water content, nuts have excellent storage qualities. They can be kept fresh for many years in sealed containers provided they are stored in a cool dry place.

ALMOND

Botanical Name: *Prunus amygdalus*
Indian Name: *Badam*

Almond is known as the king of nuts. It is highly nutritious — rich in almost all elements needed by the body. It is an effective health-building food, both for the body and mind, and a valuable remedy for several common ailments.

There are two varieties of almonds, the sweet and the bitter. Among the sweet variety are the thin-skinned and thick-skinned ones. The thin-skinned, known as *kagzi* in India, is the superior one. The bitter variety should be avoided as these almonds contain prussic acid, a poison. They have, however, commercial importance and are used for producing almond oil, perfumes and cosmetics.

Origin and Distribution: Almond is a native of Morocco. The Romans called it the 'Greek nut'. It was grown in Syria and Palestine regions during the Biblical times. It is now grown in several parts of subtropical regions, especially in Morocco, Italy, France, Portugal, California South Africa, Australia and many parts of Asia.

In India its cultivation is mostly confined to Kashmir and some areas of Himachal Pradesh.

Food Value: Almonds are amongst the best nut and seed foods. The best way of using almonds is to soak them in water and grind into fine paste of blanched almonds i.e., after peeling of the skin. This paste is called almond butter. It is easily assimilated and is preferred to dairy butter by many vegetarians. This butter is of special value for the elderly who are generally bothered with the problem of not getting enough protein in their diet. Almond butter is not only a source of high quality protein but also other food ingredients in their most easily digestible form.

Almond milk is easily prepared by grinding blanched almonds to a smooth paste and adding cooled boiled water to the consistency of the milk. With addition of little sugar, it makes a delicious and

Almonds*

Food Value		Minerals and Vitamins	
Moisture	5.2%	Calcium	230 mg
Protein	20.8%	Phosphorus	490 mg
Fat	58.9%	Iron	4.5 mg
Minerals	2.9%	Niacin	4.4 mg
Fibre	1.7%	Small amounts of	
Carbohydrates	10.5%	Vitamin B Complex	
	100%		

**Values per 100 gms edible portion | Calorific Value - 665*

nutritious drink. Upto one kilogram of milk can be obtained from 250 gms of almonds. As in case of ordinary milk, almond milk can be converted into curd and butter. Almond milk is rich in vitamins and possesses certain advantages over ordinary milk. It is more easily digestible than cow's milk and is useful for those who are not able to tolerate cow's milk.

The unsaturated fat in almonds makes it one of the most beneficial of fat. In specific terms, every 100 gms of almonds contain 11 gms of linolenic acid. This fatty acid is one of the most polyunsaturated fats and highly beneficial for lowering serum cholesterol levels.

Natural Benefits and Curative Properties

The medicinal properties of almonds arise chiefly from pharmaco dynamic action of copper, iron, phosphorus and vitamin B. These chemicals exert a synergic action and help formation of new blood cells, haemoglobin and play a major role in maintaining smooth physiological functions of brain, nerves, bones, heart and liver. Almond is highly beneficial in preserving vitality of the brain, in strengthening the muscles and in prolonging life. It forms a vital part of all tonic preparations in Ayurveda and Unani medicines.

Paste of almonds with milk cream and fresh rose bud paste applied on face daily is an effective beauty aid. It softens, bleaches and nourishes the skin. Its regular application prevents early appearance of wrinkles, black heads, dryness, pimples and keeps the face fresh.

A teaspoonful of almond oil mixed with a teaspoonful of *amla* juice, massaged over scalp, is an effective remedy for falling and thinning hair, dandruff and premature graying.

The skin of almonds should preferably be removed by soaking them in water for one or two hours before consumption as it contains irritating properties. Almonds should be thoroughly chewed and should not be eaten immediately after meals. They are a highly concentrated food, with high calorific value, and should mostly be used with bulky vegetables and fruits like raw turnips, lettuce, cucumbers and apple.

Anaemia

Almonds contain of 1.15 mg per 100 gms of copper in organic form. The copper along with iron and vitamins, acts as a catalyst in the synthesis of blood haemoglobin and therefore useful food remedy for anaemia.

Constipation

Almonds are highly beneficial in treating chronic constipation. It is an excellent laxative — 11 to 15 kernels taken at bed time facilitate a clear motion the next morning. Those with weak stomach can take seven grams of almond oil with hot milk.

Impotency

Almonds are very useful in case of low sexual energy resulting from nervous debility and weakness. Regularly eating an equal quantity of almond kernels and roasted gram helps in restoring sexual vigour.

Skin Disorders

Wild almonds are considered useful in skin diseases, especially eczema. A few leaves of wild almond are pulverised with water and the cream so prepared is applied to the affected parts. Almonds are also beneficial in treating pimples. The endocarp, which is hard cover of the seed, should be ground with water and applied over the affected parts. In case of inflammatory condition of the skin, external application of almond oil eases the pain and cools the heat.

Respiratory Diseases
An emulsion of almonds is useful in bronchial diseases, hoarseness and tickling cough. It is prepared by pounding the nuts and mixing the powdered kernels with orange or lemon juice. A teaspoonful of the oil given with 10 drops each of fresh white onion juice and ginger juice, daily thrice, for a fortnight, is useful in whooping cough, bronchitis and asthma.

COCONUT

Botanical Name: *Cocos nucifera*
Indian Name: *Narial*

Coconut is known as a 'wonder-food'. It is a near perfect food, containing almost all essential nutrients needed by the body. It is also considered a sacred fruit and held in high esteem in religious ceremonies in India. It is offered as a token of devotion while performing *pooja* in temples.

The outermost part of coconut is shining green when tender, and becomes hard, rough and matty on maturity. Coconut is covered with a thick layer of stout fibres, at times the layer is over 25 mm. thick. Then follows a hard, stone-like layer, about 6 mm. thick. The inside of this stony layer is lined with a thick coating of soft, milky-white flesh. The cavity inside the flesh is filled with a water-like fluid.

Origin and Distribution: Coconut is believed to have originated in the Indo-Malaya region and to the south west of New Guinea. There is evidence that the coconut was grown in India about 3,000 years ago. The *Vedas* describe coconut tree as *Kalpa-Vriksha* or the tree of heaven. According to Hindu mythology when Lord Vishnu, the God protector of universe, came to this earth, he brought with him the *Karpagavalli*, the coconut tree, which means giver of all health, energy, strength, tranquillity, longevity and peace.

Coconut reached East Africa, and possibly Panama before 1492 AD. Thereafter, it spread to other tropical areas of the world. It grows abundantly along the sea coasts and thrives well in loose sandy soil growing to a height of 20 to 30 m. The age of a coconut tree ranges from 80 to 200 years.

Food Value: Coconut is highly nourishing and strengthening but a fattening food. However the high oil content is easily digested and more easily utilised by the body than other fats. This oil closely resembles butter in physical and chemical properties. The protein content of coconut is of high quality, containing all amino-acids. It is also rich in potassium, sodium, magnesium and sulphur. The energy value of dried coconut is high, being 662 calories per 100 gms.

Coconut*

Food Value		**Minerals and Vitamins**	
Moisture	36.3%	Calcium	10 mg
Protein	4.5%	Phosphorus	240 mg
Fat	41.6%	Iron	1.7 mg
Minerals	1.0%	Vitamin C	1 mg
Fibre	3.6%	Small amounts of	
Carbohydrates	13.0%	Vitamin B Complex	
	100%		
		Fresh Coconut's Calorific Value - 444	
**Values per 100 gms edible portion*		*Dried Coconut's Calorific Value - 662*	

Natural Benefits and Curative Properties

Coconut is used in all stages of maturity. As a food, it is most valuable before it matures. Its jelly-like tender kernel contains various enzymes and is easily digested. Ripe kernel is rich in fat and carbohydrates. It does not have high protein like other nuts and can be taken with green salads and cooked green vegetables. It is, however, difficult to digest with starches. The milk of fresh coconut is a valuable food for children suffering from nutritional deficiency. It has a more vitamin A content than the coconut itself. It has adequate natural minerals and a high quality protein both of which are valuable for growth and repair of the body.

The water of the tender green coconut, generally known as mineral water, is used as a beverage and a refreshing drink. A fully grown and about one month old tender coconut contains about 400 to 465 c.c. of water. The water has sugar in an easily assimilable form and is an excellent tonic. The water of a single coconut contains sufficient vitamin C to meet the daily requirements. It also contains several vitamins in the B group. These are niacin, pantothenic acid, biotin, riboflavin, folic acid and thiamin as well as pyridoxin in traces. The water also contains sodium, potassium, calcium, magnesium, iron, copper, phosphorus, sulphur and chlorine.

Intestinal Worms

Coconut is an ancient and an effective remedy for intestinal worms. A table-spoonful of freshly ground coconut is advised at breakfast, followed by a dose of castor oil after three hours. The process may be repeated till the cure is complete.[1]

Acidity

The mature dried coconut is useful in treating acidity. The oil reduces the acid secretion of the stomach giving relief to the patient.

Digestive Disorder

Tender kernel of coconut is highly beneficial in treating digestive disorders like indigestion, colitis, gastric ulcers, diarrhoea, dysentery and piles. The water of tender coconut is also an excellent remedy for flatulence, vomiting and dyspepsia. In vomiting, it is of great medicinal value when other methods do not seem to work.

Dry Cough

Coconut water mixed with a table-spoonful of poppy seeds, milk and one table-spoonful of pure honey, taken every night at bedtime is an effective remedy for dry cough due to throat irritation or excessive smoking.[2]

---

1. Dr. S.J. Singh, *Food Remedies*, pp. 74, Nature Cure Council of Medical Research, Lucknow, 1982.
2. Dr. Aman, *Medicinal Secrets of Your Food*, pp. 482, Indo-American Hospital, Mysore, 1985.

Cholera

Tender coconut water is very useful in cholera. About 300 ml of this water mixed with a teaspoonful of fresh lime juice administered orally rectifies the electrolyte balance and neutralises acidosis of the blood. Coconut water is a potassium-rich fluid, and since cholera patients can almost invariably take oral fluids following initial correction of shock and acidosis, experts suggest intake of coconut water as essential for cholera patients.[1]

Urinary Disorders

Coconut water acts as a natural diuretic in heart, liver and kidney disorders such as scanty and suppressed urination, albuminuria, that in presence of protein in urine, dropsy and high acidity of urine.

Bilious Fever

Coconut water is highly beneficial in treating bilious fever. It should be given frequently in small doses. Normal drinking water should, not be taken immediately after drinking coconut water but can be taken after some time, if necessary.

Ascites

Coconut water is valuable in ascites, a disease which causes fluid accumulation in the stomach. The patient should be given two or three glassful of coconut water and the quantity increased or decreased according to the condition and the needs of the patient.

Skin Disorders

Oil extracted from the flesh of a ripe nut is an effective dressing for burns and scalds. It is of great value in ointments as it penetrates the skin readily. The tar-like fluid obtained from the red, hot shell of a ripe nut is a rubifacient which causes reddening and warming of the skin. It is a household remedy for ringworm, itch and other skin diseases.[2]

---

1. Ibid., p. 485.
2. J.F. Dastur, *Medicinal Plants of India and Pakistan*, pp. 61, D.R. Taraporevala Sons & Co. (P) Ltd., Bombay, 1985.

Uses

Coconut oil is the most important of all its by-products. It is made into coco jam, coco butter, margarine, vegetable butter and salad oil. The oil is a hair-restorer and a widely used hair oil. Dried coconut is used in cooking and in preparing of sweets and curries. The milk from a dried coconut is a good medium of cooking in place of ghee or oil.

GROUNDNUT

Botanical Name: *Arachis hypogaea*
Indian Name: *Mongphali, Peanut*

Groundnut is a legume belonging to the pea and bean family. It is, however, categorised as a nut because of its high nutritional value. That is the reason it is used in meals and snacks.

Groundnut is the only nut that grows below the ground. The plant is a variable annual herb which grows upto 50 cm in height. The flowers of the plant develop a stalk which enters the soil and forms a pod generally containing two seeds. When they mature the leaves turn yellow and the plant is removed from the ground and dried. After three to six weeks they are separated from the plant.

Origin and Distribution: Groundnut is a native of South America. In the 16th century, the Portuguese took it from Brazil to West Africa and the Spaniards took it across the Pacific to the Philippines. From there, it spread to China, Japan, Malaysia and India. India leads the world in groundnut production with about 40 per cent of the groundnut entering the world commerce is from India.

Food Value: Groundnut is particularly valued for its protein content. Kilogram for kilogram groundnut contains more protein than meat — about two and a half times more than eggs, and far more than any other vegetable food except soyabean and yeast. The proteins in groundnut are well balanced, except for slight deficiency in some essential amino acids. As it happens, these amino acids are abundant in milk which can be combined with groundnut products for better results.

For proper digestion, groundnut requires thorough mastication. Experiments with the groundnut show that it is quite indigestible unless chewed to a smooth paste. This difficulty is obviated by roasting. The baked starch increases digestibility. As an alternative to chewing, groundnut can be ground into a paste which on account of its richness in fat, is called 'peanut butter'. A little salt is generally added; some peanut oil can be mixed if it becomes dense.

Groundnut*

Food Value		**Minerals and Vitamins**	
Moisture	3.0%	Calcium	90 mg
Protein	25.3%	Phosphorus	350 mg
Fat	40.1%	Iron	2.8 mg
Minerals	2.4%	Vitamin E	261.4 mg
Fibre	3.1%	Small amounts of	
Carbohydrates	26.1%	Vitamin B Complex	
	100%		

**Values per 100 gms edible portion | Calorific Value - 567*

Natural Benefits and Curative Properties

Groundnut is one of the most nourishing foods. The U.S. Department of Agriculture considers it rich in five important nutrients — energy protein, phosphorus, thiamin and niacin.

Apart from nutritional value, groundnuts have considerable medicinal value. They contain oil which is easily digested. It is as an excellent aperient or a mild laxative and emollient which softens the skin. Eating fresh roasted groundnuts with jaggery and goat's milk is very nutritious for growing children, pregnant women and nursing mothers. It strengthens immunity, particularly against tuberculosis and hepatitis.

However, excessive use of groundnuts can cause acidity, spermatorrhea and premature ejaculation. Some individuals are allergic to roasted groundnuts. Asthmatics in particular should abstain from eating excess of groundnuts; Groundnuts boiled in salted water are a better and less harmful option for such individuals. Liberal use of groundnuts should also be avoided by persons with gastritis and jaundice; excessive use causes hyperacidity, indigestion and heartburn.

Obesity

Experiments show that weight can be reduced by eating a handful of roasted groundnuts with tea or coffee without sugar an hour before lunch time. It reduces appetite and leads to gradual weight less.

Diabetes

Groundnuts are valuable for diabetics. Eating a handful of groundnuts daily prevents malnutrition, particularly deficiency of niacin, and checks development of vascular complications.

Diarrhoea

Groundnuts are also useful in diarrhoea, especially chronic diarrhoea. This type of diarrhoea is caused by nicotinic acid deficiency. Groundnuts contain required quantity of niacin which is valuable in controlling this problem. Patients can benefit greatly

Groundnut Milk and Groundnut Curd

Groundnuts can also be used for preparing nutritive and tasty milk. About 500 gms of lightly roasted nuts are soaked in water for two hours, the skin removed by rubbing in water and the nuts ground into a fine paste. The paste is mixed with water three times its bulk and strained through a fine sieve. This milk can be safely boiled without loss of food value. In nutrition and composition, groundnut milk is similar to dairy milk and may be used as its substitute.

Groundnut milk can also be made into curd. A small quantity of the cow-milk curd is added to the milk and allowed to remain overnight to set. It tastes like normal milk-curd and possesses much of its qualities.

by drinking goat's milk with lemon squeezed alongwith a handful of fresh roasted groundnuts.

Teeth Disorders

Chewing fresh groundnuts with a pinch of salt strengthens gum, cures stomatitis, kills harmful bacteria and safeguards teeth enamel. The mouth must however, be rinsed with water after eating groundnuts.

Beauty Aid

A teaspoon of refined groundnut oil, mixed with equal quantity of lime juice, applied on the face daily at bedtime keeps the face fresh. Its regular use keeps the skin nourished and prevents acne.

Uses

Groundnuts may be eaten raw, boiled, steamed or roasted. They are sometimes eaten as a sweetmeat by coating them with sugar. In the West, they are often taken as nut chocolates, candies, sandwiches and other food products.

Groundnut flour is becoming increasingly popular; it is far superior to wheat flour in nutritive value.

Groundnuts are often used as vegetables when the seeds are still tender. They are also be taken in their germinated form. Germination not only makes them more digestible, but also enhances their food value, especially their vitamin B and C content.

MUSTARD SEEDS

Botanical Name: *Brarrica nigra*
Indian Name: *Rai*

Mustard is a well-known oil seed. It is a small annual plant with long intermodes, simple, alternate and soft yellowish green leaves, and grows upto a height of one metre. The fruit is a pod with seeds inside.

Dry mustard seeds are small, measuring about 1 mm. in diameter. They are round and darkish-brown or greyish-brown in colour. They have no smell, but when pounded and moistured with water, emit a pungent odour. The taste of mustard seeds is bitter and pungent.

Origin and Distribution: Black mustard is a native of Eurasia. This was the first species to provide table mustard for use as a condiment. The plant is cultivated as a field crop in most temperate countries.

Food Value: Mustard seeds are used as a condiment. The seeds yield 28 per cent of a fixed oil which is used in medicine and soap-making. The seeds also contain about one per cent of a volatile oil which is used as a counter-irritant when greatly diluted. The oil from the seeds is used in North India as a hair oil, a cooking medium and to prepare pickles and salads. In Punjab, Delhi and Western Uttar Pradesh, the leaves are used as a vegetable.

Natural Benefits and Curative Properties

Mustard seeds as well as its oil is used in many quasi-medical prescriptions. White mustard seeds can be beneficially used as a beauty aid. A handful of these seeds are roasted in a litre of sesame or coconut oil, the oil strained and cooled and applied with little water over face before going to bed. This cures pimples and whitens the complexion. Mustard oil boiled with henna leaves is useful in promoting healthy growth of hair. About 25 gms of mustard oil should be boiled and a little quantity of henna leaves gradually put in this oil till about 60 gms of these leaves are burnt. The oil should then be filtered through a sieve and stored in a bottle. Regular head massage with this oil promotes hair growth.

Poisoning

Mustard seeds have emetic properties which cause vomiting. A teaspoonful of seeds, mixed in a glass of water, generally produce free vomiting in five to 10 minutes. This is especially useful in drunkenness, narcotic poisoning and other similar cases of poisoning.

Muscular Pains

Mustard is a rubefacient which causes reddening and warming of the skin. A plaster or paste made with water, is applied as analgesic in rheumatism, sciatica, paralysis and other muscular pains. The plaster should, however, not be applied directly to the skin but a layer of lint material put between the mustard paste and the skin. Direct application may cause painful blistering.

Convulsion in Children

A teaspoonful of powdered mustard seeds mixed in about five litres of warm water is used as therapeutic bath in convulsions caused by high fever in children.

Ringworm

Mustard paste is highly beneficial in treatment of ringworm. This paste is applied after washing the skin with hot water.

SAFFLOWER SEEDS

Botanical Name: *Carthamus tinctorius*
Indian Names: *Kusum, Kusumbha, Karadai*

Safflower is an important oil-seed crop. It is a highly branched, glabrous, annual plant, with long and stout taper roots, and dark green, glossy leaves. Florets are tubular and usually orange-yellow coloured. Safflower seeds are bitter in taste and look more or less like the seeds of orange.

Origin and Distribution: Safflower is believed to have originated in an area bounded by the eastern Mediterranean and the Persian gulf. It was initially cultivated in Egypt, the Middle East and India for the orange dye obtained from the florets, a dye which is still used. Safflower was taken by the Spaniards to Mexico. It was introduced experimentally as an oil crop in United States in 1925, where it is now grown on a commercial scale.

In ancient Sanskrit literature safflower has been described as *kusumbha*, from which the common modern name of kusum is derived. *Kusumbha* oil was regarded as purgative and identical properties were assigned to it in Egypt, Africa and India.

Food Value: Oil content of the seeds varies from 20 to 38 per cent. The thinner the hull the greater is the oil content. The oil has a high linoleic acid content, about 75 per cent, and a very low linolenic acid content. The crude protein content of the expressed meal or cake varies from 20 to 55 per cent, depending on the amount of hull removed during processing.

Natural Benefits and Curative Properties

Safflower oil is one of the most polyunsaturated oils. The medicinal value of linoleic acid came into prominence in the 1960s following publication of a series of research findings in medical and scientific journals that this fatty acid was highly beneficial in lowering serum cholesterol levels in laboratory experiments. From virtual obscurity safflower oil became a bestseller within a few years.

It has also now known that linoleic acid promotes and improves availability of calcium to the body's cells, thereby virtually acting as a vitamin. Some scientists refer to it as "vitamin F".

Heart Disease

Safflower oil has proved beneficial in lowering blood cholesterol and can be used liberally by persons suffering from cardio vascular disorders.

Constipation

One teaspoonful of kernel of the seeds taken with six shelled almonds and honey has proved highly beneficial in the treatment of constipation. It is a safe laxative for the young, the weak and pregnant women. A popular Unani medicine called *Jwarishe Qhurtum* is prepared from safflower seeds.

Sexual Debility

Safflower seeds are highly beneficial in treatment of sexual debility. Powder of dry seeds mixed with pistachio nuts, honey and almonds and taken with milk before going to bed is a very effective aphrodisiac; it improves sexual vigour and thickens semen.[1]

Asthma

Safflower seeds are highly beneficial in treating bronchial asthma. Half a teaspoon of powder of the dry seeds, mixed in a tablespoonful of honey, can be taken once or twice with great benefit. It acts as an expectorant and reduces spasms by liquefying the tenacious sputum. Infusion of the flowers mixed with honey is also useful.[2]

Female Disorders

A decoction prepared by boiling two teaspoonfuls of powdered seeds in 120 ml of water is given as a remedy to cure painful menstruation. Dried flowers mixed with rose is also given as a medicine in this condition. A brew made from safflower foliage is said to prevent abortion and female sterility.

Eczema

It has been established in animal tests that eczema can result from lack of linoleic acid. Safflower oil can thus be beneficially used in the treatment of this disease. Two tablespoonful of safflower oil daily is advised; the quantity can be reduced to one tablespoonful as the condition improves.

SESAME SEEDS

Botanical Name: *Sesamum indicum*
Indian Name: *Til*

Sesame is a well known oilseed and probably the oldest of all cultivated seed crops. Since the ancient times it has been regarded as a food of high value in Asian societies.

1. Hakeem Mohammad Musa, *Random Notes*, pp. 180, Urdu MS. Kachiguda, Hyderabad, 1901.
2. Dr. Aman, *Medicinal Secrets of Your Food*, pp. 520, Indo-American Hospital, Mysore, 1985.

Sesame is a variable annual herb, one to two metre tall, covered with glandular hairs and with a somewhat foetid or pungent smell. The seeds are small, smooth, white, red or black.

Origin and Distribution: Sesame originated in Africa. It has been identified in the excavation at Harappa, Pakistan, dating to 2000 BC and was recorded in Egypt about 1300 BC at the time of the expulsion of the Israelites. The seeds and oil are widely mentioned in Indian literature of the Vedic period and both the seeds and the oil are used for religious ceremonies such as *shraddha* and *pitryana*. It spread early through West Asia to India, China and Japan.

Food Value: Sesame seed kernels make a nourishing food. The hard husk of sesame seeds must be removed prior to consumption; it acts as an abrasive on the intestines and due to its high concentration of oxalic acid. The husk is rich in calcium, iron and vitamin B_1, but these are unfortunately non extractable by human digestive system.

Natural Benefits and Curative Properties

There are three varieties of sesame seeds — black, white and red. The black yields the best quality of oil and is also best suited for medicinal purposes. The white seeds are extremely rich in calcium and useful in case of calcium deficiency. The red variety has an exceptionally high iron content. The seeds are an emollient that softens the skin, are a nourishing tonic, an emmenagogue that stimulates menstruation, a demulcent, laxative, diuretic and fattening.

The oil extracted from sesame seeds is of high medicinal quality. Charak, the great medical authority of ancient India, has said that of all oils, the gingelly or sesame oil is the best. It has the finest flavour and a high boiling point. This latter quality is important from health point of view, for it indicates that less molecular restructuring takes place in sesame oil than any other seed oil.

Piles

Sesame seeds are highly beneficial in treating piles. They can be taken in the form of decoction or as sweet-meats. Ground to paste with water, they are given with butter for treating bleeding piles.

Skin Disorders

A poultice of the sesame seeds can be applied externally over ulcers, burns and scalds; application of a mixture of equal parts of sesame oil and lime water is also effective. The oil is also used as a substitute for olive oil in pharmaceutical preparations for external uses.

Anaemia

Black sesame seeds, with their rich content of iron, are valuable in anaemia. An emulsion of seeds mixed with a cupful of milk and sweetened with jaggery, should be given to patients suffering from anaemia. This emulsion is prepared by grinding and straining the seeds after soaking them in warm water for a couple of hours.

Dysentery and Diarrhoea

Sesame seeds are useful in dysentery and diarrhoea. Two tablespoonfuls of lightly roasted seeds are ground into a fine powder and mixed with one tablespoon of cow's ghee. This mass is divided into three parts and each part is taken with boiled goat's milk thrice a day for six days by patients suffering from chronic dysentery or diarrhoea. It acts as an excellent medicine in these conditions.

Abortion

Sesame seeds have traditionally been used for abortion. One tablespoonful of the seeds ground with equal quantity of palm jaggery and used twice daily in the early stages of pregnancy causes abortion.

Respiratory Disorders

The seeds are valuable in respiratory disorders. An infusion of sesame seeds, mixed with a tablespoonful of linseed, a pinch of common salt and a desert spoon of honey, should be given once at night in case of acute and chronic bronchitis, pneumonia and asthma. It acts as an expectorant.

Menstrual Disorders

Half a teaspoon of powdered sesame seeds taken with hot water twice daily reduces spasmodic pain during menstruation in young anaemic unmarried girls. Its regular use, two days prior to the expected periods, cures scanty menstruation. Warm hip bath containing a handful of bruised sesame seeds should be simultaneously taken along with this recipe.

Hair Disorders

A decoction of crushed leaves and root used as a hair wash is said to treat dandruff, premature greying and promote hair growth.

Uses

Sesame is grown for its edible seeds which are the source of gingelly oil. This oil is used as a substitute for olive oil both in salad dressings and in cooking. The fried seeds are taken in soups and, mixed with sugar, are a popular sweetmeat in Africa and Asia.

SUNFLOWER SEEDS

Botanical Name: *Helianthus annus*
Indian Name: *Suryamukhi*

Sunflower seeds are probably the most familiar of all edible seeds; they are found in the tightly packed core of sunflowers. The flowers are large in size, yellow in colour and always facing the sun. There are many varieties of sunflower seeds. The larger kernels are generally used for edible purposes while the smaller for crushing into edible oil.

Origin and Distribution: Sunflower is believed to have originated in the Mexican region. It was introduced in Europe in the 16th century, where it became popular as an ornamental flower but was recognised as an oilseed crop in Eastern Europe. The first commercial production of oil began in mid-nineteenth century. The crop steadily grew in importance and soon became one of the world's most important oilseeds.

Food Value: Sunflower kernels contain above average protein, apart from phosphorus and iron concentration and are a rich source of B-complex vitamins.

Sunflower seeds can be used to enrich any meal. They can be sprinkled over cereals, salads, yogurt and soups and mixed with vegetables to augment protein, vitamin and mineral content. They can be used in desserts and can be taken as snacks between meals.

Natural Benefits and Curative Properties

Sunflower seed kernels can be considered as complete food. Taken with milk, the seeds contribute protein, the substance of which every cell of the body is made. The kernels contain almost 50 per cent fat which makes them a highly satisfying food and prevents any feeling of fatigue, of being run-down and weariness resulting from intake of too much carbohydrate and sugar.

Being rich in potassium, the seeds help balance the sodium in our diet, thereby protecting the body from the dangers of too much salt in body tissues. Magnesium being plentiful in sunflower, helps the heart and other muscles as well as nervous tissues in maintening a proper balance between magnesium and calcium.

High Cholesterol level

The seeds contain substantial quantity of linoleic acid which is helpful in reducing cholesterol deposits on the arterial walls. Substituting solid fats like butter and cream in the diet with sunflower seeds therefore, leads to great improvement in health.

Beriberi and Pellagra

As a rich source of thiamin and niacin, sunflower seeds help protect the health of nerves, the brain, the skin and the digestive tract. Lack of these vitamins produces deficiency like beriberi and pellagra.

Anaemia

The flour of sunflower seeds is one of the richest sources of iron and highly beneficial in preventing and treating anaemia.

Respiratory Diseases

Powder of dry seeds or decoction of pounded seeds is used as a remedy for bronchitis, laryngitis, tonsillitis, influenza and cough. There is a belief in some parts that growing sunflower in the home garden prevents influenza and cold.

CURD

Botanical Name: *Yogurt*
Indian Name: *Dahi*

Curd or yogurt is a lactic fermentation of milk with a smooth, pleasant and refreshing taste. It is one of the most valuable of therapeutic foods — highly versatile and health promoting.

Cow milk is generally used for preparing yogurt in Europe and North America whereas in India buffalo milk is mostly used. In Russia it is the milk of sheep, goat and mare which is largely used for the same purpose.

Pure milk should always be used for making curd. Before it is curdled, the milk should be boiled for about 10 minutes and the temperature of the milk brought down to a lukewarm range. Freshly cultured starter is then to be added and mixed thoroughly with the milk. Generally one teaspoonful of starter is sufficient for every 500 ml of milk.

To a great extent the quality of curd depends on the starter used. The better the starter or the seed, the sweeter is the aroma and firmer the curd texture. In hot season milk curdles easily but in cold season becomes is necessary to cover it with a blanket and keep it in a warm place. It generally takes about six to eight hours for the milk to coagulate in hot season; in cold weather it takes 12 to 16 hours for it to form a firm mass.

Origin and History: Curd has played an important part in diet of practically all societies. From time immemorial it has been and continues to be regarded as a wholesome food the world over.

Food Value: Curd is a highly nourishing food. It is a valuable source of protein, essential vitamins and minerals. It is also a rich source of calcium and riboflavin. The protein in curd is more readily digested than milk protein. It has been estimated that regular milk after an hour being taken is only 32 per cent digested whereas 91 per cent of curd is digested within the same period of time. This makes it an ideal diet for those with sensitive digestive systems, particularly young children and elderly persons.

Natural Benefits and Curative Properties

Although curd has a nutritive content similar to fresh milk, it is of special value for therapeutic purposes. During the process of making, the bacteria converts milk into curd and predigest milk protein. This bacteria inhibits the growth of hostile, illness-causing bacteria in the intestinal tract and promotes good bacteria needed for digestion. The good bacteria facilitates absorption of minerals and aids in the synthesis of B group vitamins. Buttermilk,[1] has the same nutritive and curative value as curd.

Curd is considered one of the best aids for natural radiant looks. It supplies the nerves and the skin with healthy ingredients and counteracts the ill-effects of exposure to the scorching sun. The bacteria in curd makes the skin soft and glowing. Curd mixed with orange or lemon juice is a good face cleanser. It supplies moisture to the skin and the fruit juice provides the essential vitamin C. One tablespoonful of juice should be mixed in one cup of curd and applied to face and neck, allowed to dry for 15 minutes before wiping with a soft tissue and washing with water.

A mixture of oatmeal flour and yogurt has been also found effective in making the skin fairer and softer. This mixture should be applied on the face for 15 to 20 minutes and then washed with warm water. For pimples, a paste of curd and Bengal grain flour or *besan* should be applied on the face and then washed off.

Curd*

Food Value		**Minerals and Vitamins**	
Moisture	89.1%	Calcium	149 mg
Protein	3.1%	Phosphorus	93 mg
Fat	4.0%	Iron	0.2 mg
Minerals	0.8%	Vitamin A	102 IU**
Carbohydrates	3.0%	Vitamin C	1 mg
	100%	Small amounts of Vit B Complex	

**Values per 100 gms edible portion | Calorific Value - 60 | **Int'l Unit*

1. Buttermilk is prepared by churning curd and adding some water, removing the fat in the form of butter.

Curd is a valuable hair conditioner — for softer, healthier and stronger hair. It should be massaged into the hair roots before washing. Dandruff can be removed by massaging hair for half an hour with curd which has been kept in the open for three days.

Gastro-intestinal Disorders

Curd brings relief from gastro-intestinal disorders such as chronic constipation and diarrhoea. Apart from the lactic acid organisms placed in the milk for the purpose of souring, the acid of sour milk and its lactose content are important factors in curing a number of diseases.

Orla Jensen, author of *Lactic Acid Bacteria*, observes that yogurt and fermented beverages can be frequently used in case of gastric irritation when other foods cannot be retained by the stomach. The lactic acid is completely metabolised to carbon dioxide and water and is not excreted in the urine. It also does not have any effect on acid-base balance in the system. It is an alkaline food. Besides aiding digestion, curd decreases dryness and gas in the stomach by helping in secretion of hydrochloric acid, pepsin and renin.

The germs which give rise to infection and inflammation (such as those which cause appendicitis, diarrhoea and dysentery), cannot thrive in the presence of lactic acid found in the curd and buttermilk. Beneficial results have been achieved by using buttermilk in cases of colitis. Buttermilk enemas have been found beneficial in the

The Legend of Curd

It is believed that curd was first made in Turkey. Legend has it that while travelling through a desert, a nomad kept some milk in a goat-skin bag and hung it across the back of his camel. On opening the bag few hours later, he found that the liquid has transformed into a thick tangy delicious custard. The desert sun and the bacteria inside the bag had produced the necessary conditions for preparation of yogurt.

treatment of colitis, chronic constipation, diarrhoea, dysentery, chronic appendicitis and gastric ulcer.

Premature Ageing

Curd has been associated with longevity. Prof. Élie Metchnikoff, a noble prize-winning Russian bacteriologist of the Pasteur Institute says that premature ageing and decay can be slowed by taking sufficient quantity of curd as part of daily diet. He made an intensive study of the problem of old age in the early 20th century and came to the conclusion that the normal human diet acts like a slow poison and weakens immunity. This process can be arrested and the intestinal tract kept healthy by constant, regular use of yogurt or some variety of acidophilus milk.

Hepatitis/Jaundice

Excessive liberation of ammonia, one of the major causes of coma in hepatitis, can be prevented by liberal intake of curd. The lactic acid organisms in the curd counteract the formation of ammonia. In jaundice, curd or buttermilk sweetened with honey, makes an ideal diet.

Burning in Rectum

Severe burning and itching in the rectum after passing stool can be controlled and successfully treated within days with liberal use of curd and lemon juice and bland diet. Curd makes the stool acitic and alleviates the burning and itching sensation.

Skin Disorders

The use of curd in the form of buttermilk is highly beneficial in treating obstinate skin disorders such as psoriasis and eczema. The application of buttermilk compresses is useful in these conditions. Pads of muslin or thin cloth saturated with buttermilk may be applied to the surface. The compresses may be worn continuously or only at night. The surface should be properly cleaned when the compress is removed. These compresses are very effective in case of skin inflammation. The intense skin irritation generally disappears after the application of buttermilk compresses.

Uses

Curd is used in numerous ways in Indian culinary. It is eaten with both meat and vegetable curries, with rice, fruit and fish, eaten plain with salt and pepper, or with sugar, honey, fruit, molasses and with innumerable essences. Many dishes are cooked in curd. It is also extensively used as buttermilk and *lassi*. Over 50 per cent of the total milk in the country is converted into curd.

HONEY

Indian Name: *Shahad*

Honey is a highly prized gift of nature. It has unique nutritional and medicinal properties. It is a viscid, saccharine substance, semi-translucent of a light yellowish-brown colour. It has an aromatic odour and sweet acrid taste. After some time it becomes opaque and crystalline. Bees alone are capable of making honey and honey comb.

The word "honey" is derived from the Arabic "han". This became 'honing' in German and 'huning' in old English.

Origin and History: In India, honey has been used for several thousand years as an ingredient for medicines. In Egypt it formed the basis of numerous medical preparations. Hippocrates, the father of medicine, prescribed it as a remedy for several ailments. He believed that honey combined with other foods was nourishing and health-giving. Aristotle, the father of natural science, held that it improved health and longevity.

It is well known that the ancient Egyptians and Greeks used honey to embalm their dead. It has a wonderful keeping quality. In a tomb of one of the queens of Egypt who was buried over 3,000 years ago, a jar of honey was found without any appreciable change in its chemical composition. It has been recently found that honey can retain all its qualities for over two decades.

Food Value: The sugars in honey are glucose, fructose and sucrose. Glucose is the simplest of the sugars. It occurs in the blood of live animals, in fruit and vegetable juices. Its restores the oxygen that is replaced by lactic acid when fatigue sets in. Fructose, which is also known as levulose or grape sugar, crystallises more easily than glucose and builds up tissues. Sucrose is a combination of glucose and fructose. Dextrin, a type of a starchy fibre, is found in small amounts in honey, which makes it more digestible.

Research indicates that the pollen in honey contains all 22 amino acids, 28 minerals, 11 enzymes, 14 fatty acids and 11 carbohydrates. Unfortunately much of the nutritive qualities are lost when honey is heated to 150°F for commercial use. The process of filtering, bottling and cooling to protect its flavour, removes the pollen grains and does not leave the honey as a pure product.

Honey*

Food Value		**Minerals and Vitamins**	
Moisture	20.0%	Calcium	5 mg
Protein	0.3%	Phosphorus	16 mg
Minerals	0.2%	Iron	0.9 mg
Carbohydrates	79.5%	Vitamin C	4 mg
	100%	Small amounts of Vit B Complex	

**Values per 100 gms edible portion | Calorific Value - 319*

Natural Benefits and Curative Properties

Honey is one of the finest sources of heat and energy. Energy is generated mainly by carbohydrates and honey is one of the most easily digested forms of carbohydrates. Because of its dextrin content it enters directly into the bloodstream thus providing almost instant energy. It is a boon to those with weak digestion. All body organs respond favourably to honey. The famous Roman physician, Galen, has described honey as an all-purpose medicine for all types of diseases. It is now used as a curative and preventive for several ailments.

One spoon of fresh honey, mixed with juice of half a lemon in a glass of lukewarm water and taken first thing in the morning, is an effective remedy for constipation and hyperacidity. Fasting on honey-lemon juice water is highly beneficial in the treatment of obesity without any loss of energy and appetite.

A mixture of honey and alcohol is believed to promote growth of hair. It is said that Japanese geisha girls with their luxuriant hair, mix several tablespoonful of honey with alcohol and massage it onto the scalp, allowing it to remain for two hours before rinsing with shampoo. They claim that regular use of honey-alcohol mixture stimulates hair follicles to grow into luxuriant tresses.

Heart Diseases

Dr. Arnold Lorand, an eminent nutrition expert considers honey as one of the best foods for a healthy heart. He observes, 'Honey is easily digested and assimilated; it either prevents flatulence or does not cause it. I strongly recommend it in cases of arteriosclerosis and weak hearts. As it would be unwise to leave such a hard working organ as the heart without food over the long hours of the night, I recommend heart patients to take a glass of water mixed with honey and lemon juice before going to bed'.[1] Honey is useful in cardiac pain and palpitation of the heart.

Anaemia

Honey is remarkable in building haemoglobin largely due to its iron, copper and manganese content. It is beneficial in treatment of anaemia; it helps to maintain the right balance of haemoglobin and red blood corpuscles.

Pulmonary Diseases

Honey is highly beneficial in the treatment of lung diseases. It is said if a jug of honey is held under the nose of an asthma patient and inhaled, the breathing becomes easier and deeper. The effects last for about an hour or so. It is the mixture of vapour of 'higher' alcohols and ethereal oil which soothe and benefit asthma patients. It usually brings relief whether the air flowing over the honey is inhaled or whether honey is taken in milk or water. Some authorities recommend one year old honey for respiratory diseases.[2]

---

1. Ibid., p. 23.
2. Ibid., p. 37.

Skin Diseases

Applied externally, honey, is considered useful in the treatment of wounds and sores. Dr. N. Zaiss, a leading Austrian physician before the World War, claimed to have successfully treated thousands of cases of wounds, sores and ulcers with honey. According to him honey, soothes pain, acts as an antiseptic, hastens healing and is especially effective in curing burns and carbuncles.[1]

Irritating Cough

As a demulcent or a soothing agent, it has a soothing effect on the inflamed mucus membrane of the upper respiratory tract and relieves irritating cough and symptoms like difficulty in swallowing. For the same reason, it is used in the manufacture of various cough mixtures. Honey gargles are useful in irritant cough.

Insomnia

Honey is beneficial in treatment of insomnia. It has a hypnotic action in bringing sound sleep. It should be taken before going to bed, in doses of two teaspoonfuls from a large cupful of water. Babies generally fall asleep after taking honey.

Oral Diseases

Honey is valuable in keeping the mouth healthy. Applied daily it cleans and sparkles the teeth and keeps the gums healthy. It prevents tartar deposit and prevents decay and early falling. Being a mild antiseptic, it prevents the growth of harmful micro-organisms. In case of ulcers in the oral cavity, honey helps in early healing and prevents further sepsis and pyogenic infection related bad odour and pus formation. Gargling with honey water is very useful in gingivitis resulting from inflammation of the gums.

Eye Diseases

Honey is an excellent remedy for various eye ailments. Applied daily in the eyes, it improves the eye-sight. It is very useful in the treatment of itching of the eyes, trachoma, conjunctivitis and other similar diseases. Its regular internal as well as external application prevents glaucoma in initial stages of the disease.

---

1. Ibid., p. 35.

Honey is valuable in preventing cataract formation. Two grams of a mixture of onion juice and honey applied locally to the eyes with a glass rod is an effective remedy for immature cataract. It resolves the already coagulated protein fibres as well as prevents further coagulation.

Diseases of Stomach

Honey tones the stomach, helps in proper digestion and prevents stomach problems. It decreases the over-production of hydrochloric acid thereby preventing symptoms like nausea, vomiting and heartburn. Honey acts as a laxative and emetic and clears putrified faecal matter and undigested foods present in the alimentary canal.

Old Age

Honey is especially useful in providing energy and heat to the body in old age. It dries the phlegm and clears the system of mucus generally seen in old age. One or two teaspoonful of honey in a cupful of boiling water, taken warm, is a refreshing and strengthening drink.

Sexual Debility

Honey is a spermatogenic and a sexual stimulant. It is regarded by many Asiatics as an aphrodisiac. They believe that it possesses a magical substance which influences both fertility and virility. In ancient days, a simple honey potion was said to offer a feeling of rejuvenation. It was prepared by boiling three parts water to one part honey over a slow fire until two thirds remained. This honey potion was believed to promote a feeling of rejuvenation and youthful virility.[1]

---

1. Carlson Wade, *Health Secrets from the Orient*, pp. 208, Allied Publishers Pvt. Ltd., Bombay.

MILK

Indian Name: *Doodh*

Milk is considered as "nature's nearly perfect food." It is also is one of the most common foods. It occupies a unique position as a health and healing food.

Cow, buffalo and goat milk has been used from times immemorial. In some regions milk of sheep and mare is also used. Cow milk contains almost twice as much protein as human milk and less sugar. Buffalo milk contains more fat than cow milk.

Food Value: Milk is regarded as a complete food. It contains protein, fat, carbohydrates, vitamins, various minerals and all ingredients considered essential for sustaining life and maintaining health. Milk protein is of the highest biological value and contains all amino acids essential for our body. A litre of milk provides all the calcium needed by an individual for one day, practically all the phosphorus, a liberal amount of vitamins A and C, one third or more of the protein, one eighth or more of iron, at least one fourth of the energy, and some vitamins B, E and D.

Milk ranks high in digestibility. The cow milk fat is 99 per cent digestible, its protein 97 per cent and its carbohydrates 98 per cent. Milk is said to require about one and a half hours for digestion. It curdles almost immediately after reaching the stomach. The organic salts and water are absorbed almost immediately while the solid matters are passed into the intestines where the fat is quickly absorbed by the lacteals.

Milk*

Food Value		**Minerals and Vitamins**	
Moisture	87.5%	Calcium	120 mg
Protein	3.2%	Phosphorus	90 mg
Fat	4.1%	Iron	0.2 mg
Minerals	0.8%	Small amounts of Vit B Complex	
Carbohydrates	4.4%	K and P	
	100%		

**Values per 100 gms edible portion | Calorific Value - 67*

Natural Benefits and Curative Properties

According to Charaka, father of the Indian system of medicine, milk increases strength, improves memory, removes exhaustion, and promotes long life. Experiments have amply corroborated Charaka.

Milk is well accepted as a wholesome food for persons of all ages, from infancy to old age. It is of special value in feeding infants, toddlers, growing children and expectant and nursing mothers. It is also recommended as a wholesome food for invalids.

Under Weight

Milk diet is highly beneficial in increasing body mass and weight. If one is considerably below the normal weight, the there will be gain of upto one to two kgs a week, depending upon the quantity of milk consumed. The body will gradually fill up, eyes will become clear and bright and the complexion will assume a healthy glow. The assimilative organs gain renewed energy and power and there is permanent weight gain.

Poor Blood Circulation

An exclusive milk diet is very valuable for those suffering from poor circulation. The natural increase in circulation results from increased amount of fluid assimilated by the stomach and intestines. Hands and feet, which are usually cold in case of poor circulation, become warm, feel alive and the patient gets a feeling of well-being within a few days of being on milk-diet.

Hyperacidity

Milk diet is very effective in cases of hyperacidity and other acid related conditions of the stomach. As milk is rich in alkaline forming elements, it quickly relives acid conditions of the system.

Insomnia

A glass of milk, sweetened with honey daily at bedtime is advised in treating sleeplessness. It acts as a tonic and a tranquilliser. Massaging milk on the soles of the feet has also been found effective.

Respiratory Disorders

Milk has proved useful in respiratory disorders such as common cold, hoarseness laryngitis, tonsillitis, bronchitis and asthma. A glass of pure boiled milk, mixed with a pinch of turmeric powder and few broken pepper, taken at night for three nights yields beneficial results.

Skin Disorders

Cream of milk mixed with a little vinegar and a pinch of turmeric powder makes an effective dressing for cuts, wounds, other simple traumatic injuries and eczema. It also makes an effective poultice in healing blood boils and wounds without sepsis.

Beauty Aid

Milk is useful as a cosmetic and a beauty aid. A fresh lime squeezed in a glass of boiled milk left for 10 minutes and regularly applied over hands, arms, face, neck and soles at night and allowed to dry, before washing with warm water the next morning whitens complexion and makes the skin soft. Washing hair with milk and egg yolk every day promotes hair growth and protects scalp from diseases.

SUGARCANE

Botanical Name: *Saccharum officinarum*
Indian Name: *Gannā*

Sugarcane is the most important member of the plant kingdom with a metabolism leading to accumulation of sucrose. It is transported as glucose and fructose within the growing plant. The crop provides the cheapest of energy-giving food.

Sugarcane is a perennial plant which grows from 2.5 to 4.25 metres in height. The diameter of stems varies from 2.5 to 8 cm. It has several joints after every few centimetres.

Origin and Distribution: Sugarcane is indigenous to India. It has been cultivated since the Vedic period and is mentioned in several ancient scriptures. The names sugar and sugarcane have been derived from the Sanskrit word, *sharkara.* Alexander and his army carried sugarcane to Europe around 325 BC. India is amongst the top sugarcane growing countries; others being Brazil, Cuba, China, Mexico, Pakistan, the U.S.A., South Africa and Columbia.

Food Value: Juice extracted from the cane is nutritious and refreshing. It contains about 15 per cent natural sugar and is rich in organic salts and vitamins.

Sugarecane juice is a refreshing soothing drink on hot summer days. A little lime juice added to the juice improves its flavour.

Natural Benefits and Curative Properties

Sugarcane juice strengthens the stomach, kidneys, heart, eyes, brain and sex organs.

Sugarcane*

Food Value		**Minerals and Vitamins**	
Moisture	90.2%	Calcium	10 mg
Protein	0.1%	Phosphorus	10 mg
Fat	0.2%	Iron	1.1 mg
Minerals	0.4%		
Carbohydrates	9.1%		
	100%		

**Values per 100 gms edible portion | Calorific Value - 39*

Fevers

The juice is beneficial in fevers. In febrile disorders which cause fever leading to protein loss sugarcane juice supplies the body with necessary protein and other food elements.

Genito-urinary Disorders

Sugarcane is very useful in scanty urination. It keeps the urinary flow clear and helps the kidneys function properly. It is also valuable in burning micturition due to high acidity, gonorrhoea, enlarged prostate, cystitis and nephritis. For better results, it should be mixed with lime juice, ginger juice and coconut water.

Jaundice

Mixed with lime juice, sugarcane juice can hasten recovery from jaundice. It is, however, essential that the juice be hygenically extracted, preferably at home. Resistance is low in hepatitis and any infected beverage can make matters worse.

Weak Teeth

The juice sucked from chewing sugarcane is highly valuable in strengthening teeth weakened by excessive use of soft foods. Chewing to suck sugarcane juice exercises the teeth, makes them strong, keeps them clean and increases their life.

Thinness

Rapid gain in weight can be achieved by drinking sugarcane juice regularly.